ACCIDENTAL ADDICT

A True Story of Pain & Healing....

also *Marriage, Real Estate, and Cowboy Dancing*

LINDA CREW

For Madeline Rubin, MSW LCSW

She listened.
She believed the things I told her.
She helped me hang onto myself.

And as always, of course, for my husband, Herb

He stubbornly maintained his faith in me
even when, over and over,
I insisted I could not possibly go on.

For I am fearfully and wonderfully made.

Psalm 129:14

FOREWORD

I am well. Completely well.

Wonderful.

Except, I'm lying.

Or was the first time I wrote this, anyway.

Month after month, on days when I felt optimistic enough to imagine that surely I was nearly healed, I watched myself nail this story down on faith alone that by the time you'd read these words, they'd be true.

And now, thank God, they are.

I am completely, confidently well.

It feels like a miracle.

It almost feels like I've been dead, and now I've come back to vibrant life.

I was a happily married mother of three grown children and the author of nine novels, most of them for young readers, all but one brought out by large New York publishers.

In September of 2012, I optimistically presented myself for total knee replacement surgery—one of 670,000 such patients in the U.S. that year—and, thanks to doctor–prescribed Oxycodone and Xanax, promptly descended into three years of drug-induced hell.

My addiction and recovery did not involve any wildly out-of-control, pop-star type behaviors. No flipping out in public, no speeding cars. No brushes with the law at all, in fact. I did not wind up in prison, being interviewed for *20/20* by Diane Sawyer. I never assaulted anyone. I didn't steal. I never even told a lie. The only gun involved is the one I repeatedly imagined needing, the one I'd next day thank God I'd not had close at hand.

I do not flash back to traumas of my childhood. There *weren't* any. My parents loved and nurtured me. They stuck my four-month-old toes in the sand at my grandparents' beach cabin in Yachats. They took me camping at lakes in the Cascades and towed me on water skis behind their motor boat on the Columbia River. The whole thing was probably as close to *Leave it to Beaver* as real life ever gets.

People sometimes fake their memoirs. You've heard that, right?

Not me. Congenitally consigned to tell the truth, I can't bring myself to make scenes worse than they were, salting in exaggerated bits of movie-ready violence, nor can I embellish with whatever images might be uplifting—the popular near-death, light-at-the-end-of-the-tunnel scene, for example—much as I, along with everyone else, enjoy reading such narratives and do so hope they're true, do feel dismayed whenever an author is forced to admit they're not.

Every scene I describe actually happened. If I were to claim I'd been aboard a helicopter taking fire over Iraq, for example, I'd be able to back that up (!) I've changed a few names, but no one depicted is a composite character. These are the actual health care professionals I encountered, a few of whom may come to wish I'd been handing out a card: **Warning: Anything you say to this person will be remembered.**

Because it will. That's how I am. Even while I was assuming my brain was too far gone to ever again write another book, I think the observer in me never stopped mentally processing all this as *story*.

Sometimes a writer assigns herself a challenge of experience, deducting her expenses on Tax Form C, then reports back, allowing the reader to decide for herself whether she'd like to embark on some rigorous diet, raise chickens in the backyard, divorce from all screens, sample a new fitness craze, or travel to some trendy eco resort.

This book is no such thing.

No one would ever choose to experience what I and so many others have gone through in suffering withdrawal from physician-prescribed drugs, but since my life took this horrific turn and I happen to be a writer, it feels like being tapped on the shoulder—Tag, you're it. Speak up.

Stories of addiction-related depravity abound; explanations of how people eventually recover, not so much. Mine is the story I longed to hear during my withdrawal: a story of hope, solid evidence that people *can* somehow live through this and survive. If you read this book some years in the future, rest assured you need not fear Googling my name only to find that I relapsed right after its publication. Whatever lies ahead for me, one thing remains certain: I will not be going down in the flames of ongoing addiction.

Because of the powerfully destructive effects of narcotic painkillers and anti-anxiety benzodiazepines on the brain, I was, for the duration of my prolonged healing, a terribly sick, reclusive woman, in certain stretches nearly comatose and, in my bleakest moments, the raging Bitch of the World.

Ask my family.

Here's how it all went down—the white, middleclass, "nice-lady," pharmaceutically-induced trainwreck of my life.

CHAPTER 1

My trees are probably wondering where I've been all this time.

I'm afraid the answer's not pretty.

But on this gloriously spring-like day, with rare-for-January sunshine streaming in low from the south, I'm finally feeling good enough to head out and check on them. *Let's just see how far I can get,* I think, using the sort of encouraging self-talk in which I've recently developed such proficiency. *Let's just see what will happen if I try acting like a healthy, confidently energetic person.*

Out in the driveway at the pick-up's tailgait, I press in my ear-buds and dial my iPod to the playlist my husband made as background music for a novel I was working on three years ago when the little boat of my life got completely blown out of the water. I pull on my rough leather work gloves and seize the grips of the long-handled red loppers from the truck's bed, flipping the tool over my shoulders to carry as a triangle. As I saunter off toward the trees, Garth Brooks starts singing "If Tomorrow Never Comes."

My favorite trees are the Douglas firs, the far five acres Herb and I planted together almost twenty years ago now, but today I stop short, figuring to give some attention to the pines, mainly so I can work in the full, healing light, these trees not yet having gained enough height to form a sun-screening canopy.

I wade into the winter-dead weeds and start attacking the prickly hawthorn shoots; those and, as always, the wickedly arcing blackberry vines that threaten to take over the entire twenty-five acres every time I turn my back. I can't believe how young and dumb I was forty-one years ago when the Realtor showed us this place and all I could think on the subject of blackberry brambles was the endless supply of pies I'd be baking up for my darling new husband. Too much in love to see straight, I guess, and starry-eyed with Jesse Colin Young's song "Ridgetop," where he extolls the joy of a yard full of bushes that turn into pies in July.

At each pine I nip off the lowest limbs. At a dead one, I pull the roll of hot pink flagging tape from my vest pocket and tie a piece around a browned branch, a message for Herb: **Chainsaw needed here**.

The iPod playlist has worked itself to my personal, watch-what-I-can-do theme song, Maria Muldaur belting out "I'm a Woman." (Aint nothing I can't do!)

Hey, don't look now, but my positive self-talk is *working*. I am *back*. Not only that, I'm on a roll. I've *missed* this, the warmth of the sun on my shoulders as my thoughts float free. It's a laboring that smells good, too—the Christmassy scent of the sap.

Working my way north toward the golf course abutting our property, I'm so pleased to feel like myself again that it almost seems like it's okay, what I've been through. I can put it to rest. I can be forgiving. The past doesn't matter, as long as I'm loving my *now* and I actually have a decent looking future.

I clip a little pine, Alison Krauss singing, "Country Boy." I love the song, but I can never listen to it without thinking that poor guy ought to just go ahead and *ask* that prettiest girl in town to marry him. How can he be so sure she won't say yes if he hasn't got the guts to speak up?

I look up, scanning for my next tree. I never restrict myself to any rigid system of working up one row and down another. Where's the fun in that? I'm not an employee here. I'm the boss of myself and these are my own trees. I'm pretty sure that in my happy, haphazard way, I have, over time, met and dealt with each one personally.

It happens just as Alison hits the part about silver in the stars and gold in the morning sun: I trip on something and, in a twisting motion, pitch forward.

Even as I'm going down, I'm already whimpering my pathetic plea to the universe: *Do-overs?* Lying flat on my back, clenching against the pain in my right ankle: *Do-overs, do-overs.*

Hey. It's worked in the past. I once brought down a big fir limb that felled me with a smack hard enough to my shin to raise a lumpish bruise that lasted for months. I remember lying there that time murmuring *Do-overs, do-overs,* and when the pain subsided, I got up and kept working.

So for a moment I cling to the faint hope that the incantation will magically save me. Maybe it's too soon to go all Worst Case Scenario. Maybe the pain will stop.

It doesn't.

Well, shit.

I can't believe this.

Except that I can. It's *exactly* the sort of thing that would happen to me. I swear, my whole life has been blessed/cursed with dramatic good luck/bad luck timing.

I lie there looking up at the blue sky. *Oh, shut up about that poor wimp of a country boy.* I yank out my earbuds. Now I can hear a tractor over on the golf course.

Okay, let's see…my father broke his ankle in his sixties walking in a local woodland park. Son Will broke his ankle on the soccer pitch at fourteen. Stories I'll be needing to re-visit. And wait… my friend Maggie Chang suffered a broken ankle just as she was trying to pack up her household in a move from Williamstown, Massachusetts, to Bainbridge Island, Washington.

Stories. Isn't that what we always want? Something happens to us and suddenly we want to hear how it all turned out when it happened to somebody else. Our brains run a search and retrieve for the details which flew right past us upon first hearing, but which now have such sharply personal relevancy.

I push myself to sitting. Maybe I'm jumping the gun. Maybe it's not broken and I'm still suffering from hyperalgesia. Learned all about that nasty business the hard way when I was in opioid withdrawal. Here's the deal: basically, anything that's going to hurt will hurt a whole lot more. If that's the case now, it could be weirdly good news. It might mean the physical damage isn't as bad as the pain level makes it seem.

Should I pull off my rubber boot to check it out?

I briefly contemplate the boot's faded pattern of twining flower vines. Nope. Forget it. Too much trouble. And I'd just have to get the darned thing back *on*. It wouldn't solve anything. I'd still be sitting here, more up close and personal than ever before, I believe, to the winter-smelling mud. I'd still have the same problem—how to get myself back to the house.

Of course any sensible person would simply pull out her cell and call for help. And I *would* be that sensible person if I weren't so busy being the stupid person who has drowned three cell phones, one after another, never learning from my mistake, every time carefully following the same fatal procedure, throwing my Carthartts in the wash with the phone in the "handy" phone pocket, *sensibly* making sure I immediately got any residual poison oak oil washed off the pants.

My smart phone plan had been to be smart and not put the poor little device at risk. My decidedly unsmart and unfancy phone is back at the house, safely tucked in the cozy leather pocket of the Frye bag Herb wanted to buy me at Nordstrom on our way to the Bonnie Raitt concert.

Well, dammit.

I look at my watch. That's right, I'm so old, I still wear one. 11:15.

It's a five-minute, stop-start struggle to get myself upright. *Let me be happily surprised*, I pray as I brace myself with my hands. Let's say the way this goes is that my ankle feels stronger than the pain is suggesting.

Nope. As usual, I'm not calling the shots on this story. I'm just trying to live it. This is an ankle that doesn't want any weight put on it.

I stick the loppers point down in the mud and begin a labored sideways perambulation, taking a little hop to the left, using my right foot only for glancing balance. Hardly efficient. My left knee is artificial as of two-and-a-half years ago and, oddly, one maneuver that just doesn't seem to work after knee replacement is hopping.

Ten minutes of this tedious business gains me about ten feet, just over an old irrigation pipe and into the grassy, slightly less bumpy road that divides the pines from the poplars. To my left I see a tractor pass on the golf course a hundred yards away, but I no sooner entertain the thought of yelling for help than I abandon it. Too many memories of chasing Herb down in field, forest, or orchard, yelling for attention, silently begging for him to just, please, for God's sake look up and see me. But when men are engaged with their roaring machines—tractors, mowers, chainsaws, whatever—they don't look up. They're not supposed to.

I turn right, toward the house, recalling stories of people crawling incredible distances from accident sites with broken limbs. I'm picturing hands and knees, though, and that's another thing artificial knees don't do well. Only when the whole ordeal is over will it occur to me I might have made better time scooting backwards on my rear, using my ever strong triceps to haul myself along. In the middle of it, though, with the ground so boggy, I don't think of it. Besides, it's taken me so long to stand myself up, the idea of trying to get back down would hold scant appeal.

Painfully slow going, each tiny hop and wincing drag, but I see no alternative. Herb watched me go off towards the woods with such enthusiasm earlier that he wasn't necessarily expecting to find me at the house when he came home around 12:15. He said if he wasn't there when I came up for lunch, I should figure he'd gone back to the grocery store. If I lower myself onto the damp turf and simply wait, my rescue might not come for hours.

I look at my watch again when I reach the grassed-over road along the river. Thirty minutes. Oh, man. At this rate I'm risking missing him entirely. I just *have* to make it into earshot before he drives up.

Suddenly the Bible verse read at our wedding comes to mind: *Two are better than one, for they have a good reward for their labor. And woe to him who is alone when he falleth, for he hath not another to help him up.*

No shit.

Alan Berg, former mayor of our town and a Unitarian minister, read those selected words right there in the front yard of the very house I'm trying to get back to now. Standing under the oaks in my home-sewn, Victorian, $65-in-materials wedding gown, I certainly never envisioned four decades later having to demonstrate this *nobody to help me up* bit quite so literally.

Yeah, woe to me.

The ditch I hopped coming out must now be sloshed through, the business end of the loppers sinking into the mud, the brown water soaking the hems of my Carhartts. Ten minutes more and I can finally see the battered old mailbox where the road ends, our driveway taking off on the other side.

I've just required a full hour to manage the distance I covered in three minutes going out.

Back in that oh-so-briefly happy life.

It's 12:15. Herb should come driving up any minute. He won't look this way, I know it, so I won't waste precious energy trying to flag him. I'll just listen carefully and wait until I hear him park up by the house, get out of the car and slam the door. Then I'll start yelling.

Okay, I hear it. A vehicle.

But, no, it's the Fed-Ex truck. Never mind, same plan. Help is help.

Suddenly I realize. We've all seen it in the movies a million times, but I've made it my entire life so far without ever having to shout out that call for assistance. Not in this anonymous way, hoping a stranger will hear.

It's hard, somehow. Oddly embarrassing. I mean, really, how stupid of me to be unable to keep an operating cell phone handy. And is there an actual category for being accident prone? My lifetime record has obviously now edged over the line into the officially ridiculous.

I watch the guy shoulder a long package—probably fruit trees Herb's ordered—and swivel for the porch.

Well, nobody's ever accused me of being shy about speaking up; now is not the time to start.

"Help!"

A plane's roar drowns me out. Damn. Obviously the guy doesn't hear me.

I wait until I can see him again at the back of his truck.

"Help! Out here!" I stand on my least lousy leg and thrust the red loppers up in a waving motion.

He stops and looks. He's heard me. But then he turns his back, goes for the driver's side door.

Oh, come on. Seriously?

Right. I have one more chance. I hear a hint of anger in my own insistent plea because really, isn't it about time I caught a lousy break?

"*Help!*"

CHAPTER 2

Somebody was screaming. Me.

Middle of the night, nurses gathered—murmuring, fiddling with my drip lines.

Pain, brutal and overpowering, crushing me into a whimpering mess. Should I ask them to call my husband, my mother, my daughter? But they'd all gone home to Corvallis. I was alone in this Springfield hospital. And this was just—well, really, when was the last time I'd been reduced to this—crying because something hurt so bad I couldn't help it?

"Is everybody having this much trouble?" I whimpered, knowing all the patients in this wing had just been through the same thing, either hip or knee replacement surgery.

"Everybody's different," a nurse said.

Oh. So....nobody else raising hell. Nobody else shrieking in shocked outrage. I'm the squeaky wheel. The one getting the grease.

Various meds were tried in my IV line. Time. More time. Time impossible to gauge or measure. Still the pain. Nothing worked. No relief.

Grimly funny. My punishment for pride? For going into this knee surgery halfway cocky? People who'd been through it predicted pain. What, I should tremble in fear? You couldn't make me. You couldn't scare somebody like me who'd already been through plenty. Seven previous knee surgeries, two C-sections and three broken arms. Oh, and a bunch of stuff to do with infertility. Ever heard of an endometrial biopsy? Neither had I until I felt the knife.

But this. *This...*

Okay, I remembered now. My own fault. I'd been aware, through the post-surgery anesthesia haze, of family members at the foot of my bed: my mother, brother, sister-in-law. Alarmed by a wave of nausea, I'd waved them out, determined to salvage the bit of dignity I might claim by at least not vomiting in front of anybody.

"It's the pain meds," a nurse explained, adding something to my IV line. "This'll help."

"Just give me the Tylenol from now on, then," I said, remembering what I'd learned in some previous health crisis, that nausea can be worse than pain. Opioids could be bad for you anyway, it was rumored. Steer clear, all the better.

Mistake! Now I was paying. Nausea was *not* worse than this. And I'd "let the pain get on top of me," something we were warned in our pre-op classes we must never do. We must take our meds in order to be able to withstand the all-important rehab exercises that would give us nicely functioning new joints and make us candidates suitable for featuring in the glossy brochures of healthy, active post-op patients!

An angel nurse, a light in the darkness, stood holding my hands, murmuring a visualization of escaping the pain. Maybe somebody (me?) had told this shift I was a good candidate for trying to put my own brain to work for me.

Finally, something shut me up. Must have been some sort of opium derivative running warmly into my veins, because when I left the hospital, my husband was entrusted with a written prescription for Oxycodone, tablets of 5mg, one or two to be taken as needed every four hours.

Hello darkness, my old friend.

For awhile, it seemed, Oxycodone *was* my friend.

Hillbilly Heroin, my son Miles cheerfully informed me.

All three of my grown kids seemed halfway amused: Mom on drugs. Very funny.

But those pills were the number one thing on my pain-clouded mind. Herb's too. Because what happened when I slipped between doses wasn't one bit funny.

The first night home I screamed awake in the middle of the night just as I had in the hospital. Herb scrambled for the pills, holding the glass of water, trying to talk me down. He would set the alarm from now on. No going through *that* again.

He brought our laptop to the dining room table so I could do email; I was weeks from being able to crutch/climb the stairs to my office. Next to it he set the flowers our son Will had sent.

I tapped out upbeat notes to friends: **All's well, nurses couldn't have been nicer, Herb's taking great care of me, so glad to have the surgery behind me and I'm sure to be up and around soon…**

And then the hospital load of narcotics drained away and I fell, like Alice into the rabbit hole.

I lay on the chaise under the trees in the backyard. Something was clicking in my chest. What *was* that? Hours later I figured it out. Silly me. Birds chirping. But then the next day, an even weirder realization: the clicking was in my own ears, the same old tinnitus that had arrived the previous spring with a suspected viral infection.

"My brain's playing tricks on me," I complained to Herb, and asked again if it were time for my next dose of Oxycodone.

"Not quite yet."

He kept a vigilant account in his chicken-scratch scrawl. Not a single pill one minute early, but never late, either. The horrible bridge-hour preoccupied us, the toughing-it-out time before my next dose. My pain and his helplessness against it—wicked combo.

At sixty-one, I turned out to be the youngest in our class of joint-replacement patients gathered in the hospital conference room a couple of weeks before the surgery. The other women my age introduced themselves as the daughters, the caretakers for the parents who'd arrived in wheelchairs.

Oh, the daughters. What would people do without them?

According to hospital policy, in order to be discharged directly to home, a patient had to show proof of a caretaker/coach willing to sign on 24/7, for ten full days. Without that, you went to a rehab facility.

I looked around. No question, I had the best deal going. On the line of the form that asked about your coach, I wrote: **Husband, Herb Crew.** And, for good measure: **Lucky me!** We had notebooks. Like school! And school I could do. I would get an A. In fact, I planned to be the Poster Girl for Rapid Knee Replacement Recovery and Rehabilitation. When my surgeon predicted I'd be dancing again eight weeks after surgery, I joked I'd send him a post-op shot of myself in my tribal belly dance get-up to grace the cover of one of the sports clinic's pamphlets.

The instructor emphasized the importance of taking our meds right before our rehab exercises. A great deal of attention was given to the unfortunate constipating effects of the opioid pain meds and how we might take measures to combat this. We were sternly warned about the dangers to our livers of taking too much Tylenol. We learned about walkers and crutches and when we might hope to graduate to a cane.

A cane! Surely she was talking about these other people, these old people. Not me. I had a bad knee, yes, something I'd had to deal with ever since I'd knelt on a sewing needle at the age of fifteen. But I had walked in here under my own power. In the past weeks I'd repainted the interior of our Neskowin beach house on my own, and our driveway at Wake Robin Farm was still strewn with saw horses and cans of paint remover where I'd been stripping and refinishing an antique door to go into a cabin we were about to build on one of our forest properties.

I was a woman with energy.

Me? Knocked flat? Needing a cane? No way!

Knowing how wiped-out patients are going to be after surgery, how disinclined any of us would be to do anything but lie there, the clinic had insisted we book our first rehab appointment at the time surgery was scheduled. We were to show up at the local physical therapy establishment of our choosing on the fifth day after surgery.

Fifth day, period, even if you wound up being discharged from the hospital only the day before.

I hardly remember the first time Herb hauled me over there, I was so groggy. Sharon, the therapist, said this first visit was mainly about getting me up and out of the house. As far as the pain and the pills, she was talking to Herb, not me. I overheard the phrase, "Keep her comfortable."

Herb doled out my pain meds on a precise schedule, and busied himself setting up my in-home rehabilitation plan.

I'd be lying on the chaise in the backyard and he'd come out with his accoutrements—a straight-backed chair, an antique carom board, a soccer ball, the notebook with photographic depictions of the prescribed exercises—reminding me it was that time again.

He helped me to the chair and put the carom board under my stockinged feet. Then he'd push back on my left foot, sliding it along the board, urging me to tolerate just a bit more bend in my knee, a wince more pain. I'd take a deep breath, summoning strength, shut my eyes and push. Thank goodness Herb was doing the counting, keeping track of what came next; it was enough for me to just clench my teeth and try. Because this stuff hurts. These exercises are what people mean when they repeat the oft heard refrain: *Rehab is a bitch.*

But I had Herb Crew for a coach.

"That's great. That's amazing! You're doing really really well."

Because of my husband, for me, the pain would not be what I'd remember. I'd remember how I ate up this verbal encouragement. I'd heard Herb talk like this to the little girls he coached on our daughter Mary's soccer team, but he had never, ever talked like this to me. No exaggeration: this man delivered more verbal encouragement to me in those weeks than I'd heard from him in the previous thirty-eight years we'd been married.

Whatever else happened on *My Health Journey,* as the hospital's notebook so optimistically titled this little picnic we were having, I knew I'd always look back on at least this little bit with great fondness.

The first time my son Miles and his wife Ziwei came out to the farm to see me after the surgery, I sarcastically remarked how great I knew I looked puffed up with the twenty extra pounds of water weight they'd pumped into me at the hospital.

Miles's eyes went wide with a laugh. "That's a relief. I mean, to hear that's why you..."

"Look so fat?"

"Well, in the hospital I just thought, wow, is that how Mom looks without makeup?" He made a face. "Yeah....."

Thanks for sharing, honey.

I adore this firstborn son of mine, who, for the record, was the model for nine-year-old Robby Hummer in my middle-grade novel, *Nekomah Creek.*

After his drawn out and awkward adolescence, I have still not quite gotten over how goodlooking he is now, at thirty-three. Also, he's brilliant. For a living, he translates complex medical, legal and political tracts from the characters of Chinese into impeccable English. He has a heart of gold. As Ziwei puts it, he's too nice to live in China, her homeland. Once, in Beijing, he terrified her by inviting a stampede as he opened his wallet in full view of a bus station crowd, fishing out cash for some poor old lady in a wheelchair. People mobbed them. Ziwei was not amused.

His one flaw, which all who love him forgive, is his lack of subtlety in communication. His honest thoughts, suitable or not, have a way of popping right out of his mouth. Unlike his younger brother Will, he has no conception of the uses of flattery. On the good side, this means I do have one cherished memory of a time where this worked in his—and my—favor.

Opening his bungalow door to me, without preamble, he'd made my day:

"Oh my God, Mom! You look so young in that leather jacket."

"Yeah?" I blushed happily. "It was Mary's. She gave it to me."

"Ziwei! Come here and see how young my mom looks!"

Okay, since that might be it for the rest of my life, I'm hanging on to it.

Usually it seems to me that, as Miles's mother, I have somehow been designated the person he most enjoys correcting and contradicting, especially in front of other people. But that he loves me I have to believe. I'm his mom, right? I'm entitled to make that assumption, our family not notoriously torn apart by gross dysfunction? And I'm quite accustomed to the way he is. I've learned not to equate love with having the manners to throw wide the door and insist his mother step inside when she's standing on his porch.

In the months to come, though, as my brain wallowed in a sickly wash of doubt, I would lose my firm grip on this belief.

Mary and William—twins—arrived six-and-a-half years after Miles. Between the births, I was busy dealing with several knee surgeries and a clinical depression, followed by two years of escalating doses of the fertility drug Clomid. Finally, a single series of husband-administered shots of Pergonal resulted in this two-for-the price-of-one miracle.

William, the predicted boy, his tiny penis having been spotted on the ultrasound, was born first. Mary, the longed-for daughter, was the thrilling surprise.

"Look at the big eyes on this one," I heard the nurse say.

My daughter is one of my absolute favorite people on earth. Picture the face of Keira Knightley on a pint-sized Ellen DeGeneres, hands in jeans pockets, bouncing in sneakers. And no, unfortunately, the lovely face and soulful eyes are not by way of me, but rather from Herb's mother, who died when Herb was just fourteen.

After my surgery, Mary and her wife Jaci brought two T-shirts, one emblazoned with the slogan **TODAY IS MINE** and the other, **KICK SOME BUTT.** Jaci had knitted orange leg warmers. Perfect! I expected to be rocking these at the gym very soon.

I emailed my friends. **Please come visit!** If I were to survive these interminable afternoons of pain, I'd need the distraction of female chitchat. **Just talk me through this, please. Tell me your latest stories.** Herb wasn't supposed to leave me alone, so to even get to the grocery store, he needed wife-sitting backup.

One friend of thirty-three years brought her ever-upbeat attitude and a bag of gifts. From it I pulled the recent copy of *American Bungalow.*

"Marsha! I can't believe this! Honestly, I was just lying there thinking of this very magazine."

Isn't the best part of a spot-on gift the recognition that you are *known?* Marsha and I had met when our oldest children were newborn. We had shared over the years both the stories of our growing families and our interest in houses, remodeling, and redecorating projects.

It was this dear friend who, over lunch one day, told me something important about myself.

"Linda," she said, "you're a person who just has to have a project going. You're not going to be happy unless you do, and that's all there is to it."

Not that it was some amazing insight that I *enjoyed* being creative. I had demanded sewing lessons on the machine at the age of five, and I remember twisting idly on the school playground swing one recess, wishing I could just go home. I had assigned myself the making of fancy queen dresses for all my dolls, and I wanted to get busy.

What Marsha made me see, though, is that I didn't just like projects—I *needed* them.

"I wish you could explain this to Herb, though," I remember telling her. "He thinks it's his job to always be holding me back."

My mom came to visit, saying she'd just been on a winery tour. She presented a bottle of pinot gris.

"Um, thanks. But you know I can't drink at all while I'm on these meds, right?"

"Then save it for celebrating when you go off," she said. "It'll give you something to look forward to."

One friend stayed chatting long enough to distract me past my four o'clock dose of Oxycodone. By the time she left and I was crutching my way to the back porch, my teeth were chattering.

Herb came out to meet me.

"I need my...my...." Wordlessly distraught, I showed him my shaking arm.

"Oh, jeez." He got me in on the bed, hustled to fetch the meds. "Guess I should have brought these to you, but out the window you looked like you were doing okay."

I swallowed the tablets, lay there with my eyes shut tight. *Kick in. C'mon, kick in.*

Looking back, if I could watch this on video, I'd be hitting pause. *Would somebody please clue these people in?*

Because this was just ten days after surgery. Yes, my knee ached, but the widespread body pain and violent shaking went beyond the effects of surgery. This was the first sign: Oxycodone had its hooks in me. I was already suffering from inter-dose withdrawal.

CHAPTER 3

It's no trick to imagine enjoying being waited on hand and foot, but nobody wants to need it, not if they've had firsthand experience with the frustrating reality.

I was forbidden to take a step without two crutches. Forbidden to try carrying anything. "Could you bring me that book?" I'd have to ask. "No, I'm sorry, not that one. The other one."

Sometimes the temptation to try not being so dependent would get the better of me, which only annoyed Herb.

"Will you just sit down? What do you want? I'll get it for you." He wasn't about to have me falling on *his* watch.

In sickness and in health. Rough gig. Constant pain makes a person cranky. But what a challenge, trying to be patient with somebody whose face is stuck in a permanent wince and what she's got to say is never pleasant.

I felt for Herb.

One afternoon, getting up from the backyard chaise, struggling with my crutches, I fell.

"Jesus Christ!" Herb was beside me in a second, but not fast enough to stop me from twisting down.

I lay on the grass, eyes shut tight, as if opening them would make this real. *Do-overs, do-overs.* Because **Fall** is the number one item on the list of **Things NOT to do in your first days post-op.**

"I think I'm okay," I said, opening my eyes to Herb's worried face. "Maybe I kind of instinctively fell on my right hip."

"You didn't jerk your bad knee?"

"No." I took a deep breath. "Oh, but, I wish I hadn't done that. So stupid."

That night in bed my pain seemed worse than ever. Had I knocked something loose? Opened inner stitches? I'd avoided envisioning the details of my beat-up old knee, the surgery, and the new artificial knee too, for that matter; I really had no idea what might be going on in there. All I knew was that I was afraid, and fear was exacerbating the pain.

I asked Herb to call the clinic in Eugene. Could I maybe up my dose of Oxycodone a tiny bit?

No, the on-call doctor said. Two choices: I could go to the emergency room in Corvallis or tough it out and call the clinic in the morning.

The emergency room did not sound inviting and—funny thing—it never occurred to either Herb or me to just go ahead and knock out an extra Oxycodone tab or two. I had a fear of authority from way back, plus an almost pathological adherence to whatever rules were set before me. As for Herb, although in his life he had, at times, exhibited more of a rebellious streak than I, in this case, he was working hard at being the world's best rehab caretaker and coach. He wasn't about to be caught defying official medical advice.

So **tough it out** was our assignment. I was remembering some study showing that the act of smiling, the very activation of those particular muscles, could trigger the good neurotransmitters of pain relief.

I fell asleep that night feeling like an idiot, grinning desperately into the darkness.

I found on my To-Read stack a book long ago lent by my writer friend Margaret Anderson: *The Spirit Catches You and You Fall Down,* by Anne Fadiman. Turned out to be perfect for me in these days. A Hmong family's arduous cross-cultural quest in California to secure medical care for their beloved ailing daughter put my own troubles in perspective. At least we were all speaking English here.

The Hmong notion of physical health and a person's spirit being inextricably linked intrigued me, their interpretation that when illness strikes, it indicates the soul has gone wandering away from the body.

I could buy that. Maybe my soul had started wandering away about a year ago. I'd been experiencing some strange and, for me, uncharacteristic attacks of depression which I attributed to my fluctuating thyroid levels. But I'd no sooner get my meds adjusted and my levels stable than some new symptom would pop up. I woke one spring morning with my left ear blocked and hurried to my doctor.

I always thought my PCP Sarah Miller looked like Sarah Michelle Geller, a decade or two older, a Buffy who went to med school instead of slaying vampires. I had not been unhappy to land with her when our earlier PCP, Dr. Herrick, retired. She had once commented that many of her female patients just didn't feel right unless their thyroid test number for TSH was kept under 1.0. Since I seemed to be one of those, I very much looked forward to *not* having to argue this as I had in the past with male doctors.

Today, instead of the quick wax extraction I was expecting, she diagnosed a virus and put me on prednisone.

"People sometimes feel very energetic on this," she said. "Once in awhile somebody will actually get a bit manic."

Bingo! Check it out! That somebody was me! Turned out people were prescribed prednisone for any manner of affliction where a calming of inflammation is required. People got mad, they got sleepy, they got fat. I was the only person I knew of (other than TV journalist Jane Pauley, who wrote about it in her memoir, *Skywriting*) who enjoyed ten days of euphoria. Good thing I already had a writing project going—my memoir, *Wedding in Yangshuo*. Every morning—and sometimes in the middle of the night—I went to my office and climbed on a wild, bucking stallion that careened me around the confines of that tiny room. I wrote like a maniac. Literally. Brilliant ideas crackled along the neurotransmitters of my brain, one being the notion of placing a Chinese character at the beginning of each chapter. Family. Love. Prosperity. With lightning speed and confidence I maneuvered through Google Translate, deftly popping in one lovely character after another. How amazing and lucky and fateful that my firstborn son—he of the Big Words list in his baby book—would be able to vet all these for me, crack translator of Chinese that he's become! My God, my entire universe was falling into place! The precise and perfectly evocative words I needed shot from my brain to my fingers to the keyboard. What a revelation! You get so much more written when you're absolutely confident of your ability and you aren't wasting time berating yourself! I thought of one of my favorite books, *Bird by Bird*—something about the horror of coppery-breathed banshees at your back, taunting you with your absolute lack of any talent whatsoever. Wow! I loved how prednisone shut them right up! Damn, I better write to Anne Lamott about this!

Except...wait. Was this what it felt like to be manic-depressive? No wonder writers and artists sometimes resist the leveling drugs that take away their creative highs. I remembered a writer whose novels I much admired explaining in an interview how she'd persuaded her doctor to calibrate her meds to allow her creative energy to continue to fire its sparks. Now I understood what she'd meant. But when I ran a search, I learned to my horror that she had subsequently done a heartbreaking crash-and-burn. Maybe this euphoric state was crazily amusing, but not sustainable.

I'd been practically vibrating with assurances to Herb I was writing the most amazing book ever, bound to be published to great acclaim. After reading it, people would no doubt flock to Yangshuo just like they'd booked trips to destinations described by Elizabeth Gilbert in *Eat, Pray, Love!* Ziwei's mother would triple her bookings at her quaint little hotel! But why stop there? Seriously, why shouldn't my brilliant literary offering boost the economy of the entire region of Southern China?

Unless...oh, damn. What if I'd just written a pile of shit?

I remember the exact moment, sitting on the sofa, when this thought snaked its way into my shining happy place. **Alert! Magic meds wearing off.**

Later, Dr. Miller registered alarm when she heard all this. "Didn't you tell anybody?"

Well, I'd told anybody who'd asked; she hadn't. I told the hearing specialist she'd sent me to, although clearly he hadn't communicated with her about me, their mutual patient. I'd wondered at the time why she hadn't been concerned enough to call and ask how I'd done with the side effects of this potent drug (dynamite stuff!) but the truth is, in spite of the negative physical consequences—I hardly slept all week—I was enjoying the creative mania too much to alert her with complaints.

"You should never be prescribed this again," she warned me sternly. "I'm putting that on your chart."

"Yeah?" I pouted. "It was actually kind of fun. I finished a whole book."

Her face scrunched with skepticism. "But was what you wrote any good?"

I looked at her, offended. "It was still *my* writing." Okay, so I'd realized it was probably premature to buy the Chinese-style silk dress for the red carpet at the Academy Awards ceremony when the film version was nominated, but re-reading my work, I thought it was decent. Those were still my words, my experiences and insights. The most powerful drug in the world couldn't pull something out of a person's brain that wasn't already in there, right?

"I only ask because we had one guy who wrote a whole bunch of stuff that was just garbage, and then he never really came all the way back."

Oh. Okay, well, I guess we couldn't be taking risks like that. But maybe this showed my brain wiring was a little on the sensitive side. Maybe that's why I was reporting mood swings on variations of my thyroid levels that went unnoticed by other people.

Late spring of 2012 found me spending days on end down in our Doug fir plantation, keeping two burn piles going, dragging great rafts of long ago pruned-off and dried-out limbs first to one fire, then the other. I'd take a thermos of soup so I could stay out in the fresh air and not even have to hike back up to the house for lunch.

Sometime during the fifth day over Memorial weekend, a sharp pain stabbed my left knee and wouldn't quit.

Upsetting, given my history.

Half my life ago, when I was newly a mother, a series of knee operations had culminated in the surgeons telling me they were out of tricks; I'd have to go away and deal with the residual pain on my own. It was also discovered—too late to prevent my downward spiral into depression—that an endocrine imbalance had left me producing no estrogen at all. A thirty-year-old woman with no estrogen is not going to be a happy camper in the best of circumstances, right? I began to improve as soon as they prescribed hormone-replacement therapy, but I had fallen so deep into that pit, it took awhile to climb back out.

For three decades this much-operated-upon, kneecap-less joint of mine had served me well enough, but the memories of those surgeries and the depression were deeply embedded in me as scars of the one truly traumatic period of my life.

Now, for this same knee to be once again shooting pain to my brain was to trigger in me a definite post-traumatic stress reaction.

I phoned Dr. Miller, who had several times hinted she thought I might be a candidate for antidepressants.

"It's come to Jesus day," I told her on the phone. "Time for Lexapro."

"Really." I could tell this surprised her. I'd always been so resistant, so convinced my weird mood swings were strictly about my thyroid levels.

I specified Lexapro because I'd been on it briefly a few years earlier while I argued with a male doctor over the need to up my thyroid meds. It angered me when he said I was "probably just one of those people who needed to be on antidepressants for life." I was not! As soon as he gave in and upped my Synthroid prescription the slightest bit, I felt better, and made a point of getting off the Lexapro right away. I didn't deny it did its job, though. I asked for Lexapro by name now because at least I hadn't had any horrid side effects taking it, and no trouble getting off.

This time, I could feel the very day it kicked in. I'd been feeling completely hopeless; suddenly I was making plans to go back to those doctors in Eugene who'd operated on me before, get them to fix me up. Why fear the barbaric diagnostic tests I'd previously endured—dye shot into my knee prior to x-ray? I always remembered that room in the bowels of Sacred Heart Hospital as a torture chamber. My knee was already so compromised, the dye wouldn't disperse, and the frustrated doctor seemed annoyed at me for failing to hide the fact that his stupid needle hurt like hell. But they'd reportedly come a long way in thirty years. I could now have a painless MRI, right?

I hoped for the easy fix of a little arthroscopic tweaking. I'd had both kinds of surgeries, and to me, punching a neat little hole in your knee was nothing compared to cutting my long scar open again. But the MRI showed arthritis had finally settled in. My knee looked old, the sort of arthritic knee people these days were having replaced.

I'd been hearing the rave reviews of people who had new knees, and for the past few years the idea of knee replacement surgery had been hanging over me. Was I going to be a candidate for this? If so, should I put it off as long as possible, letting the doctors and their technologies improve, or should I get it over with while I was younger and could better withstand the surgery?

Also, we were hoping for grandkids. I wanted to be strong and healthy to help out when they started arriving.

Now the MRI showed my knee was shot. Okay, so—decision made.

"Sign me up," I told the doctor, who seemed as surprised by my alacrity as Dr. Miller had been at my finally agreeing to antidepressants. But I'm a decisive person. I figured a strong, new, pain-free knee was just the fix I needed to get me back on track toward whole and healthy.

Not that I'm claiming absolute fearlessness. I knew the stories: surgery has risks. But basically I was optimistic. These people clearly had it together. The building of the Beckham Clinic was about five minutes old, the décor soothing, every detail obviously chosen to help further a calm, healing atmosphere. The windows framed vistas of outdoor greenery. And the hospital—wow, with a massive two-story fireplace in the lobby, standing there felt like checking in for a vacation at a gorgeous wilderness lodge.

Such a contrast to my first knee surgery in Eugene at the age of nineteen. Back then I always had to wait in a cigarette-smoke-filled room two hours for every pre-and post-op appointment. Worse was Sacred Heart Hospital itself, where my forty-something roommate, also post knee-surgery, was allowed to chain smoke in our room, 24/7. When my mother and I whispered our complaint to the nurse, we were told nothing could be done, because, after all, couldn't we see this poor lady was "under a lot of stress?"

Well, those were the bad old days. Smoking was not allowed in the sparkling new hospital in Springfield, Eugene's sister city, and each joint replacement patient would be ensconced in a spacious private room. The surgery for me would be both extensive and expensive, but the doctors and my insurance company seemed to think I was entitled to this new lease on life. I felt chosen. Validated. Great medical minds had declared me worthy of this gift.

I liked my prospects and gave surgery prep my A Game, listening to relaxation tapes featuring a woman named Belleruth Naparstek daily reassuring me how the surgeons and scrub nurses would all be on my side, with solemn professionalism undertaking the repair of my knee. I could feel completely safe, placing myself in their competent, caring hands.

I was so upbeat, I saw no need to extend my course of Lexapro.

"But maybe you should stay on it through the surgery," Herb said. "What if there's one day in there where you don't feel like you're recovering as fast as you'd like? Wouldn't it be better to have the support of being on this stuff?"

That sounded prudent, so I kept taking it. In retrospect, a terrible mistake.

The Willamette Valley was enjoying an extraordinarily beautiful fall. I registered that much in the days after my surgery. The backyard was gorgeous, with golden locust leaves drifting down on the quilt laid over my legs.

Margaret emailed she imagined how incredibly frustrated I must be, to have the weather so nice and not be able to go out and work in the woods as everybody knew I loved to do.

Out in the woods? The very concept sounded like a misty fairytale memory. My setting in the backyard may have appeared golden to anyone else, but my mind had been consigned to another dim world entirely.

Torture. That's the word I was thinking about. Let me emphasize how much I hate it—the word, the very idea. Can't watch a movie where it plays any part in the plot. I can barely stand to write about it. But lying there, hurting, that's where my mind went—the nature of unbearable pain. Reprehensible and ultimately ineffective as torture may be, is it surprising the military wants to regard it as a useful tool for obtaining information? Isn't escaping pain the primal drive of any sentient creature? First before thirst or hunger, before seeking pleasure or, for humans, the inexpressible joy of loving and being loved, isn't this the first order of business?

Stop the pain! I'll say anything! Just stop it!

People were being tortured all over the world right this minute, I was sure. And they were braver than I. My pain was not born of cruelty, but kindness. An unavoidable consequence of the healing skills of the surgeon and the nurses who were diligently working to bring me back to health.

I should be grateful.

But no, I'm sorry, any emotion attached to this mind-obliterating agony could not possibly fall anywhere on the positive end of the spectrum.

My writer friends hinted I might think about writing. Maybe it would be therapeutic. My sister-in-law sent a cheery card expressing in her loopy handwriting the hope I was making good use of my "down time."

My dully functioning brain received all these suggestions and attempts at understanding with equal mystification. What were these people talking about? My only goal was to hang on one moment to the next. Working in the woods was some other lifetime. And writing? What a ridiculous idea. Wasn't it pretty clear to everybody I would never be writing again? And my sweet sister-in-law, known for always keeping her hands busy, wanting to picture me stitching a quilt, describing this as my "down time." Down time as if the conveyor belt of life gliding us from one event to the next had merely been temporarily halted for a welcome rest break.

This was more than down time. My soul had wandered away. Nobody else had the slightest idea just how far.

Hand covering the phone's mouthpiece, Herb stood by the bed where I was sobbing in frustration.

"It's Kim from Dr. Cramer's office. She wants me to put you on. I'm trying to get your meds refilled and I don't think she trusts me."

What the—? Wasn't it obvious I was in no shape to talk right now?

"She's *insisting*," he whispered. "Can't you try?"

Choking it back, I threw out my arm and took the phone, gulped a hello.

"This is Kim from Dr. Cramer's office. How are you doing?"

"Awful! I'm awful. I can't stand it!"

"Okay, you're going to have to calm down. I can't understand you."

"That's because I'm *crying*."

"Why are you crying?"

Was this woman for real? Through clenched teeth I grunted it out. "Because. I'm. In. Pain. I've never been in pain like this in my whole life and I can't stand it."

I heard her sigh. "Well, of course you're hurting. You've just had major surgery."

Like I could have somehow forgotten that fact?

"Now, look. You're already on a high dose of Oxycodone and this isn't good. You really can't be expecting to take so much of this medicine that you never have any pain at all."

Never have any pain at all? I was still just looking for one blessed moment where I *wasn't* having pain.

If there was any more to that conversation, I don't remember it. Somehow Herb got the refill. Oxycodone was so tightly controlled, it couldn't be phoned into the pharmacy. For each refill he would have to drive the hour to Eugene and pick up a written prescription.

In contrast to Dr. Cramer's assistant, I loved my physical therapist, who for those weeks served as my main contact with the outside world. Sharon was about my age and into salsa dancing. It was better with partners, she said, but her husband wasn't interested. We lamented men's stubborn lack of interest in such a fun activity, and I told her about the earthy groundedness of tribal belly dance, how it involved women of all ages dancing together, feeling empowered. How I couldn't wait to get back to it.

Sharon seemed impressed with my knee in terms of strength and balance, but I wasn't breaking any records for regaining range of motion. I constantly plied her for stories of other people's surgeries and their experience with the painkillers, uncomfortably aware I seemed to be needing higher doses of Oxycodone than others.

One day she introduced me to a woman just ten days post-op. This patient was a bit older than I and a lot more overweight, yet she already had the hundred-degree bend I had only achieved after a month. What was up with that? And when I asked her about her pain and meds, she waved it off.

"Oxycodone just made me silly, so I quit it."

"But what about the pain?"

She shrugged. "I do okay with ibuprofen."

I would hear this story again in the future—people who were actually motivated to quit opioids due to the initial negative side effects. This would be a blessing for them, long term. For myself, I still felt so overwhelmed by pain that I could hardly bother to register whether I was acting "silly."

"Did you hear that?" I whispered to Sharon, nodding back over my shoulder.

"Everybody's different," she said. "You have to stop comparing yourself to other people."

But how could I not? Every time my mother phoned she'd say, "*How* many pills are you taking?" And then I'd have to hear how my stepfather, who'd had knee replacement surgery just a couple of months after their wedding, had never complained about pain like this.

"And I don't remember him having to take all these pills," she repeatedly insisted.

So.....what? Did that make me a wimp? *I* certainly didn't know why my pain levels were so high and persistent. I'd been through dozens of experiences with significant pain in my life without ever before feeling so utterly defeated by it.

I knew she was concerned for me, but that never made these conversation any less exhausting. How could I explain to her something I wasn't understanding myself?

Herb and I so rarely do anything around town together, I used to wonder if people thought we'd split up. Our necessary parenting strategy had always been "divide and conquer." We still recall with amusement the day when, for some reason, we both showed up to collect Mary and Will after school. They regarded us with such grave suspicion. "Why are you *both* here?"

So when my husband signed me up for a temporary membership at his gym, Fitness Over Fifty, and started hauling me over there on a regular basis, these outings actually had a fun, date-like quality to them.

Herb would take me into the gym's far room and go through the same stretching and bending exercises we were also doing at home. Then we'd rotate around the room on the weight machines, bicycles, and treadmills.

One day the gym manager, a friendly young guy, came up to us.

"I want to know your secret," he said. "I've been watching how you two work together on this, and I'm having a hard time picturing my wife and me pulling it off quite so well."

Herb and I smiled at each other. We *were* a good team.

Resting comfortably.

You heard that phrase in movies and TV shows. It sounded so neutral. Banal, even. *The patient is resting comfortably.* Nothing, compared to scenes of miraculous recovery, Mathew on *Downton Abbey* rising dramatically from his wheelchair.

But now, to me, resting comfortably seemed like a state of nirvana. Because…resting comfortably? I never was; I hurt all the time.

Herb and I almost never watch TV together. He watches recorded soccer; I watch *House Hunters* while I load the dishwasher. But in an effort at comfort and distraction, he was making a point of joining me for episodes of *Parks and Rec* in the evening. I love

Amy Poehler and identify with her character Leslie Knope, the over-achieving good girl, just as I had always rooted for the smart, under-appreciated Lisa on *The Simpsons*.

I clearly remember the night after the gym manager's compliment. I was propped on the sofa and we'd blown through two or three episodes when suddenly it dawned on me. For the past hour or two, for the first time, *I had not been suffering*. Hey, maybe I'd taken a turn for the better. Never mind I was, at that moment, thoroughly dosed on Oxycodone. The absence of pain for just this brief time seemed like a great omen.

I was on the road to recovery.

But that very night I awoke with my entire left leg in a frightening spasm of pain worse than anything I'd felt up to that time.

Road to recovery? **Warning: Potholes Ahead.**

The next day I was lying on the chaise in the backyard when Herb handed me the phone. It was Kim from Dr. Cramer's office again. She'd already burned Herb's ears, now she wanted to hear what *I* had to say, apparently before we had a chance to compare notes and get straight what she assumed would be our fabricated stories.

"Dr. Cramer has asked me to call you because he feels you're taking way too much Oxycodone. You're still taking twelve tablets a day and you should be down to six."

She'd caught me an hour post-dose this time, Oxycodone totally doing its thing. I was calm.

"I've talked to my physical therapist about it," I told her, "and she doesn't seem alarmed."

"Well, of course not! What does she care? She's not the one writing the prescriptions for this controlled substance. She's in no danger of anybody checking just how many prescriptions go out of her office. I'm sure she's quite pleased with your progress. But really, are you being completely honest with her about how many pills you're taking?"

"Of course I am! I talk to her about it all the time." The assumption I was lying outraged me. Me, who can't even lie when I ought to. "If Dr. Cramer is so concerned, why isn't he calling and explaining this himself?"

"Oh, we can't be doing that," she said. "If the doctor phoned you personally, we would have to *charge* you for that."

So? Again I felt like Alice, put on the spot in Wonderland, forced to conduct a nonsensical conversation with some annoying and ridiculous character. In the context of everything else, how big of a deal was a bill for a phone consultation going to be?

"You know," I said, "we're really having trouble with the mixed messages you guys are sending. Herb and I have just been going on what we've been told, that the most important thing was to take the drugs and stay ahead of the pain so that I could do these rehab exercises."

She scoffed. "Where'd you ever hear that?"

"From you! Or the hospital, or whatever. All the notebooks and handouts and everything they told us in those classes." I couldn't believe it. Didn't she even know the rules patients were being given?

"The problem is," she said, "you're simply masking the pain."

Ha! If she meant by masking the pain I was trying to not feel it, yeah, exactly.

"Your body's trying to tell you to stop working so hard. Now I know your husband means well—"

"Don't you *dare* say anything bad about him. He's been taking the best care of me ever. I'll bet nobody else has as good a coach."

"Yes, well, you listen to me. It's high time you stopped listening to your husband on this and started thinking for yourself!"

Oh, my God. When she was through having schooled both of us, Herb and I compared notes. Since we'd both instinctively stuck to the truth, our stories in no way contradicted each other's. Which is more than we could say about the different streams of information that had been blasted at us from them.

My mother was disappointed I wouldn't commit to a few days at her family beach cabin, in Yachats, in October. She told Herb she thought I needed something to look forward to. After all, having something on her calendar has always been the sure cure for her.

Reclining there with my wrapped and grotesquely fat leg propped up, I couldn't fathom such a trip. My twice-widowed mother seemed to be forgetting that—spunky as she still was—when she and I went to Ocean Crest together, it was me hauling the bags up the stairs into the cabin. I couldn't even haul *myself* up stairs yet. How was I supposed to be helping her? Worrying about putting something on my calendar and then having to let her down was exactly what I didn't need.

I so hate to let people down that when Herb had promised, before my surgery, to accompanying his Aunt Catherine to her grandson's wedding in Los Angeles in October, I declined a plane ticket for myself. I love Herb's feisty aunt and wished I could go, but I feared having to cancel at the last minute, and knew that would make me feel even worse than begging off ahead of time.

Now I was so glad nobody was expecting my attendance. I was not the poster girl for recovery and rehab after all. I was a pathetic invalid. It was going to be challenge enough just taking care of myself here on my own.

I was painfully aware of not meeting anybody's expectations, but just how far from the mark I'd fallen hit home when Herb quietly revealed he wouldn't be going to Los Angeles for Catherine after all.

Wow. For us, the kids had always come first, and then, over several years, Herb's parents had taken precedence as he made repeated trips to Los Angeles in an effort to ease their final illnesses. A bit startling now, to finally find myself at the top of his list. Not that I liked being the neediest, but I would gratefully accept that designation if it meant he wasn't going to fly off and leave me alone as I'd been dreading.

He canceled his reservation at the lovely Channel Inn in Santa Monica Canyon:

My wife recently had knee surgery and is not recovering as quickly as anticipated, so I need to stay home at this time. I apologize for any inconvenience. I'm postponing this trip for now, but expect my wife will be able to travel with me in a couple of months, so we'll see you then.

Nice thought. Wasn't going to happen.

Herb was eager to do anything in his power to help me. He especially liked solutions which involved the diversion of an online search and the punching in of a VISA number.

"We need to get you a cane," he said.

I wasn't nice. I wasn't enthusiastic or appreciative. I guess this is how old people get—cranky—when confronted with ostensibly helpful suggestions reminding them of their infirmities. I was still stubbornly clinging to the hope of getting well fast enough to skip a cane entirely.

"But I think you're going to need this," he kept saying.

Finally relenting bought me only a few minutes peace before he was calling me in to the computer, wanting me to look on-line at the various choices.

"I want to make sure you get one you like."

"But I don't like canes at all. And I don't want to spend any time thinking about it."

I must have eventually given in and pointed at something, because in due course a cane of elegantly twisted, polished wood arrived. Even if I only used it for a few weeks, I ultimately reconciled this to myself, it would be a nice thing, someday when I was *truly* old and needed it, to put it back into service and remember it was my sweet, well-intentioned husband who'd bought it for me.

Back when we were young.

Okay, younger.

CHAPTER 4

My orthopedic surgeon, Dr. Mark Cramer, was the nicest guy ever, and although later I would feel his affability had been part of my undoing, in the beginning I loved it—the way he breezed in that first time with my files saying, "Wow! I get to operate on a one-hundred-and-forty-pound woman? That *never* happens!"

Okay, at five-foot-one, a hundred-and-forty was not a number I was proud of. Also, I did fleetingly question the appropriateness of his compliment, coming as it did at the expense of his other overweight female patients. But I confess: I did not linger long in contemplation of any kind of mental defense of them, busy being seduced as I was by the flattering proposition that he saw me as an appealing surgical candidate. When this same group had operated on me when I was around thirty, I'd felt pitifully conscious of *not* being an Olympic medalist, their preferred type of patient. I was not Mary Decker Slaney. I saw myself as a writer, mother, and co-manager of our farm; I needed a decently functioning knee. To them I was just a housewife, though, and how elaborate a rehab program did I need to get the laundry from the dryer to the bedroom bureaus? They gave me one post-op exercise, period.

Thirty years later, though, knee and hip replacement surgeries had become the bread and butter of the Beckham Clinic. Lucky me, I now represented the lucrative new demographic, patients in their fifties and sixties willing to take the surgical leap, hoping for more active senior years.

Dr. Cramer had labeled me a "highly motivated patient" at my pre-op exams, making sure I understood that it was people like me with the discipline to follow through on rehab who would have the best outcomes.

Now, waiting in his exam room for my very first post-op visit, I was nervous. And grouchy. This seven weeks had felt like an eternity, way too long for him to only now be evaluating my recovery in person. I couldn't help wondering if the clinic's protocol was a deliberate attempt to shield the doctors from having to hear from us until the worst of our pain was past. Maybe they hoped by implementing this strategic post-op scheduling, we'd all be in a more *My hero!* frame of mind by the time the surgeons first opened our exam room doors.

Not that Dr. Cramer wasn't a definite cut above our previous surgeons in the bedside manner department. In our experience, white male surgeons—the only kind whose knives Herb and I had ever gone under—tended to be brusquely efficient, no-nonsense types, proud of decisively yet delicately repairing body parts with their finely-honed scalpels, or even better, some clever little tool somebody had just invented yesterday. Any overt emotion was centered on the surgery itself. *Save us from being somebody's interesting patient* became Herb's motto after noting his surgeon's unabashed delight at the prospect of being able to try out his tiny new roto-rooter for the first time with Herb as the guinea pig.

Dr. Cramer, though, seemed like a genuine "people person."

"I hope the x-rays look okay," I said to Herb as we waited. My continuing pain had me worried. At my last PT session, Sharon had called my knee "cranky." She admitted we hadn't achieved the targeted range of motion. Was something wrong in there? Was I going to be a patient requiring what they euphemistically termed a "revision?" To me, a revision was something a writer did to a manuscript. Usually many times. In medical speak, it meant they rolled you back into an operating theatre and cut you open again.

"It's gonna be okay," Herb said.

I shifted uncomfortably in the exam room chair. "I'm afraid I'm going to be in trouble about the meds."

What if that Kim person was telling the truth about Dr. Cramer thinking I was taking too much Oxycodone? I'd been trying to cut back. I'd just logged three days at only six tablets, which was cutting in half my original doses. I was apparently still a far cry, though, from the typical, more successful patients who, according to the clinic handouts, had been **able to wean themselves from the medication during the first month after surgery.**

I had repeatedly re-read the section in the hospital handbook on Pain Medications, irrationally expecting a fresh reading to yield some insight I might previously have missed.

Expectations are that you should be off pain medication within 6 weeks. Some exceptions can be made. If your pain situation has more to do with chronic pain than post-surgical pain, you may be referred back to your primary care physician.

So, was I the exception? And how did they discern who had a problem with chronic pain and who just hurt like hell because they'd sawed off the ends of your bones? Did they intend this disclaimer as a warning that they planned to be quickly shut of you if your past medical records hinted of drug-seeking behavior?

Finally, Dr. Cramer came in apologizing, as he always had to, for keeping us waiting. Not that he seemed too down on himself about it. He was cultivating a reputation for totally involving himself with each patient, he pointed out, and apparently expected patients and staff alike to regard whatever delays resulted from his efforts not with annoyance, but rather a tolerant affection.

My x-rays looked great, he said. He briefly examined my knee and declared me way ahead of schedule on rehab.

Really? Not what Sharon had said, but naturally I liked his assessment better.

"We *have* been working really hard on the rehab exercises," I said.

"Oh, that's obvious. I'm sure you've done ten times what people usually do."

"Seriously? We only did what all the hand-outs said. Exercises twice a day at home and rehab three times a week. It's not like we did more."

"Oh, but see, most people hardly do any of it."

Herb and I looked at each other. Go figure. Who'd go through all this and then not follow the rules about getting your knee to bend again?

Dr. Cramer chuckled. "We just pick a high number so people will at least do *some*. We know whatever we say, people will do less."

Silly us. Just following all the rules. Good little kids.

"So," I said, "do you think that could be why I'm still having so much pain?"

"Could be."

"Because it's still really hurting a lot."

"I know," he said, his voice softening with sympathy. "It really *is* a very difficult surgery to recover from, and believe me, we don't like knowing our patients are in pain. We debate a lot whether we should be doing more to sort of...prepare people. Warn them. But everybody's so different. We don't want to scare people into actually experiencing *more* pain."

I nodded. I understood how the psychology of this might work. "Your nurse or whatever she is acted like she thought I was lying about the pain to get the pills, and Herb was out selling them on the street."

He sighed. "I know, and I am *so sorry* that you two had to go through this. We're working with her to get her to understand the sort of patients we have here, but she's coming from a different environment. She used to work at a pain treatment center where the main job was keeping people *off* of drugs."

"She acted like she thought I was already an addict."

"Again, I'm so sorry. I don't want you to have to worry one minute about that."

"So I'm okay on the doses I'm taking?"

"Yeah, I'm not worried about you. You're doing great."

So confident I was not an addict type. No worries about a nice lady like me.

Great. As it turns out, nice is no protection at all against opioids frying your brain.

We discussed trying hydrocodone to see if a slightly different formulation of opioids might work better. He added a prescription for an anti-nausea med just in case. Also a new Rx for the Oxycodone, in case that still turned out to deliver the most effective pain relief.

"We'll see you in six weeks," he said. "Wait here and we'll get those prescriptions for you."

I exhaled hugely the moment he was out the door. "I feel so much better!"

"Yeah," Herb said. "He really couldn't have been more encouraging, could he?"

I smiled. I'd never been high on Oxycodone, but now I was practically high on the kindness of this lovely man. His whole attitude was healing in itself. Why couldn't more doctors be like that?

A few minutes later, it was Kim of our nightmares who marched in, handing over the prescriptions. I hated even having to see her, but she'd apparently been instructed not to give us grief about my dosages.

"Now you hide this stuff, do you understand me? If you have anybody coming into your house, anybody at all—repair people, housecleaners, even your relatives—you make sure this is *hidden*. And I don't mean on the top shelf in the back of your medicine cabinet. That's the first place they'll go."

Herb and I looked at each other. This woman obviously had no idea about us, our lives. We promised we'd take care of the meds, but she seemed entirely unwilling to be reassured.

"You just don't know," she said, "how this stuff goes with people."

Well, she was right. We didn't. Did she think we were parents of addicts who'd come over for dinner, only to sneak in and raid our medicine chest? Insulting, almost. She *still* didn't believe I just needed Oxycodone because I was in pain.

Well, we had the prize, the prescription. We'd won. I wasn't going to worry about her.

Walking out, Herb checked it. "Is this right on the Oxycodone? One or two tablets every four hours?"

"That's what it was before."

"Ten mg?"

"No, it was five before. Wait a minute." I stopped on the stairs and turned to look at the written prescription. "Um, this actually *doubles* what he says I can take."

"That doesn't seem right."

"Well, whatever." I started my careful, cane-aided way down again. "I'm not going to double my dose. I'm not an idiot. I know I have to get off these eventually. But it does make me feel like maybe I could have taken more before. Like, I didn't have to suffer so much. He was so reassuring about it."

"Did you catch that bit back there?" Herb said. "I think he made a point of making her be the one to hand us those prescriptions."

"Yeah, and you could tell they'd been arguing, the way she was so mad. And she's just so...so *intense* about it."

"Well, you heard what he said. She's used to dealing with real addicts."

I would think a lot about these two people in the months to come.

They were both right; both wrong.

Mine the lousy luck to get caught between them.

CHAPTER 5

I finally started posting a To-Do list on the fridge again, disappointed in myself that I'd gone so many weeks without. Dismayingly, though, no matter what I now optimistically jotted down, the only time I'd ever leave the farm would be for physical therapy. Then, instead of whatever errands I'd intended to tack on, I'd come straight home, sick and exhausted, and crawl back into bed.

"I'm taking the sleep cure," I tried to joke to Herb, but it wasn't funny.

At bedtime, I *couldn't* conk out. The Oxycodone I needed for pain kept my brain frantically busy. Against closed lids I'd watch frenetic crowds of little people scurrying around—an animated Hieronymus Bosche painting. Only a Xanax tablet could pull closed the curtains of that irritating little show. Luckily—or so I thought at the time—I had a prior prescription. I always went to bed with special sleep-inducing music Herb had put together for me, a mix of flutes and harps and the sounds of rain falling, birds twittering. Nice try. Oxycodone completely overrode this loving attempt at a buffering soundtrack, and every night parked me in a 3-D theatre for the most horrific dreams—cataclysmic, end-of-the-world dramas played out in vivid Technicolor.

Every morning I woke up wrung out and exhausted.

Months before surgery was anywhere on the horizon, I'd accepted an invitation to publicly read from my book, *A Heart for Any Fate,* in November. Groups of writers were rotating around the state, and I chose the historic Kindst Bookstore in The Dalles as my venue because it sat smack on the Oregon Trail, near where Herb and I had conducted research for the writing of this particular historical novel.

My surgery date, September 12th, was selected for being the first available slot *after* the concert we'd booked at McMenamins Edgefield in Troutdale. We'd long had tickets and I wasn't about to miss my favorite, Bonnie Raitt. If, as the doctor guessed, I'd be dancing in eight weeks, surely by nine I could stand up and read from my own book for five minutes. But one October day I realized I wasn't going to make it. The organizers started talking about doing radio interviews beforehand. No way! My brain wasn't functioning well enough. Not to mention the travel. It was clear: I had to cancel.

Movies I could manage, though. As soon as it came out, we went to Steven Spielberg's *Lincoln.* At the end, I became aware of Herb choking up beside me. I glanced at him, then turned back to the screen. President Lincoln was dying, but I was still thinking only of the posts of some porch they'd shown right before the Appomattox surrender scene, wondering if the way they were configured was a good option for the porch on the cabin we were building.

"See, this just isn't right," I said as we crossed the rain-slick parking lot afterwards. "I need to get off the Lexapro. I don't *feel* anything. I should have been weepy at the end of that like everybody else."

"But it keeps you from feeling really bad, right?"

"I guess," I said. "But I don't like feeling so…flattened out. I can't get really happy. And I don't like how it makes me feel about sex."

"But you're fine!"

"No, I'm not," I said darkly.

"Well, you *seem* fine."

"Oh, for God's sake. Shouldn't my report on how I'm feeling on that front be the one that counts?"

"All right, all right. But just promise me you won't try going off the Lexapro until you get off the Oxycodone."

I agreed—a big mistake. But nobody was pausing the tape to point out the alternatives here. And later, nobody would be offering do-overs.

I finally made it to a couple of talks at the library, one given by an artist known for his paintings imagining the Missoula Floods that had carved out the Columbia River Gorge eons ago, the other by my brother, writer Bob Welch, who spoke about his latest book, *Cascade Summer.*

Being out in public again felt odd, and I tried not to register the alarm I detected in people who hadn't seen me in awhile. Nothing like a cane to add years to your perceived age.

At one of the talks—I cannot recall which—I spotted across the room Dr. Craig Leman, the surgeon who'd presided in the operating room after the accident I'd had at fifteen, the one that had impacted my life at every turn from that day forward.

The accident was my own doing. Already sewing my own clothes, I was cutting out a faux suede skirt and vest on the living room floor. Of course I was following the rules, taking no shortcuts with pins, instead painstakingly using a needle and thread to baste the tissue paper pattern to the fabric like a pro. At some point I stuck the threadless needle into the wall-to-wall carpet as if it were one big pincushion. Crawling around, I then unknowingly knelt on that needle, the pain making me jump to standing.

I had a babysitting job that night—three little kids. The parents didn't come home until 3 a.m., drunk, to find me wide awake and hurting, my leg outstretched. You can bet I would not be sitting for them again, not that they ever dared ask.

In the morning, my mother took me to the emergency room where we tried to explain what had happened, how it seemed like I had just knelt wrong on my knee, except that the pain was getting worse.

"Could she have knelt on a pin or something?" my mom asked Dr. Leman.

He gave her a look. "Don't you think there'd be a hole?"

And yet there it was on the X-ray, two fragments of the needle. It had gone into my knee eye first, snapping against my kneecap, the point probably remaining buried somewhere in the carpet padding.

I was wheeled into the operating room where, with me under only a local anesthetic, Dr. Leman went to work trying to retrieve those slippery little pieces.

Previously, as a sensitive twelve-year-old, I'd admired Dr. Leman's service on the hospital ship Hope. When he'd had to burn five warts off my fingertips (ouch!) I'd tearfully posited that the children he dealt with on the ship Hope were no doubt much braver than I.

"Oh, not necessarily," he said, which I always thought was so kind.

I was somehow investing the foreign poor with the moral fortitude I saw myself lacking, but he was acknowledging that pain was pain and I needn't feel guilty for noticing that a hot jab at the base of your thumbnail hurts the same whether your parents can pay the medical bills or not.

Because of this and several other encounters, Dr. Craig Leman already had hero status with our family, and there was no one my mother and I would trust more than this man to operate on my knee that fateful summer morning.

He was having a hard time of it. The needle bits were exasperatingly difficult to grasp with whatever tweezer-like surgical tool he was using. I could see the sweat beading on his forehead. Once, craning up, I saw reflected in the circular metal light over the table my knee—a big red hole. Ugh. I shut my eyes, lay back down.

My mother was keeping up a steady cheerleading chatter from over the doctor's shoulder.

"Don't worry, you're *going* on that backpack trip tomorrow!"

Well, no I wasn't. All the positive thinking in the world couldn't undo the mistake I'd made. And not going off to the Cascades with my Campfire buddies would be only the first of all the events in my life altered by the ruination of my knee. The only positive spin I would be able to put on it in retrospect was that I had not been a gifted athlete or dancer; no amazing career on stage or tennis court was cut short in the operating room of Good Samaritan Hospital that day.

After forty-five minutes of futilely chasing those fragments around the pulpy mess surrounding my patella, Dr. Leman gave up and had me knocked out in order to accomplish his mission.

I remember him at a post-op visit pointing out that I might put a dab of makeup on the scar in the future. This intrigued me. I thought teenage girls were not to be indulged in concerns of vanity. His needlework had left the old-fashioned kind of scar with the stitch dots along the sides, but it was only an inch long, nothing compared to what would be disfiguring my knee later on down the line. In any case I wasn't worried about cosmetics. I was more bothered that I couldn't seem to run quite like I had before.

My knee remained weak; it never fully recovered. Four years later, the spring I met Herb at Lewis & Clark College, it swelled up. The doctor my mother took me to back home in Corvallis diagnosed me with rheumatoid arthritis. Apparently just by looking at it.

"But wouldn't her other joints be affected?" my mother asked. "Don't you think this must have something to do with this business of her kneeling on a sewing needle four years ago?"

But this fellow was a rheumatologist, apparently incapable of looking at a swollen joint and seeing any possibility outside the realm of his own expertise. To a carpenter with a hammer, everything looks like a nail.

What a summer. My poor mother. She'd thought she'd successfully launched me. I was supposed to be working as a camp counselor in Idaho. Instead, here I was, lying around the house, required to stay off my feet, prescribed sixteen aspirin tablets a day. Was this forever? Was this supposed to heal me? My ears rang. Good thing I didn't cut myself that summer; I'd probably have bled out.

My parents hadn't argued my decision to transfer from Lewis & Clark to the University of Oregon; they'd have been hard-pressed to put together a second year's tuition for the expensive private school in any case. I showed up in Eugene that fall on crutches. What a treat, crutching my way up to the third floor of antiquated, elevatorless Deady Hall for my last required (and loathed) math class. No wonder I'd be claiming my nineteenth year as the worst of my life so far and for a decade to come.

In January, I underwent surgery by Dr. Beckham, whose name now graces the clinic itself. He had dismissed any notion of rheumatoid arthritis, and promised to fix me up by cleaning out my synovial fluid, explaining it would grow back.

Fine, except about a year later, my knee swelled up again. I was outraged. I'd already paid my dues! I had planned to be well forever. I was years from grasping the concept that if you have a problem with one body part, in all likelihood that will continue to be your weakness. You don't get to check knee surgery off your list, assuming you've earned a pass from ever having to revisit that particular joint again.

This time Dr. Beckham removed my kneecap, a procedure they'd not be nearly so quick to perform thirty years later, doctors having observed in the interim that without that crucial fulcrum, patients lost forty per cent of the knee joint's strength, no matter how hard they worked at muscle-building rehab.

But I did have six trouble-free years before stooping in the gravel drive at Wake Robin Farm to pick up a fallen branch, tearing the meniscus in that same forever-compromised knee, setting myself up for several subsequent surgeries and the concurrent depression.

Dr. Leman had always been aware of these operations. My mother swam at the city pool with his wife. People's stories got around.

Mom and I had always wondered if a decision on his part to put me under anesthesia immediately in order to retrieve the sewing needle might have made a difference in my outcome. It certainly seemed clear that whatever happened in those forty-five minutes on the operating table had set me up for chronic trouble.

And yet neither of us ever for one minute blamed him. Anesthesia has risks; I assume he'd tried to spare me those. If any of us were going to be blessed with hindsight, I'd have warned myself not to stick that needle in the carpet in the first place.

Now, as the library talk ended, Dr. Leman spotted me with my cane and approached. We exchanged pleasantries. He asked about my mother. Inquired about the cane. I told him I'd had total knee replacement surgery.

He listened, nodding kindly. And then he said something that utterly astounded me.

"I've wondered so many times over the years," he said, "if all your knee troubles had anything at all to do with that original accident you had with the sewing needle."

Anything at all? How about *everything*.

But such a dear man.

This would be the last time I would ever see him.

CHAPTER 6

I didn't know what to expect from Dr. Cramer when we showed up for my twelve-week check-up. After my first pre-op check, he'd sent me a letter apologizing "for the treatment you received when calling for pain medications." He reaffirmed that I was doing very well and was definitely "ahead of schedule" on healing.

He'd been so reassuring about my dosages of Oxycodone that I'd stopped worrying about cutting back. I was just trying to stay reasonably comfortable, and averaged about 50 mg a day for the week preceding the twelve-week check-back.

Mostly I wanted to find out why I was so tired. Could I be anemic? A nurse friend of ours had suggested that possibility, and seemed surprised I hadn't been prescribed iron supplements post-surgery.

"Anemia would be highly unlikely," Dr. Cramer said, when he finally came into the exam room and I brought this up. "Anyone would look at the records of the drug load you've been taking and assume that was the cause."

"I'm going in for a thyroid check tomorrow at home anyway. Would it hurt to do an iron check too?"

"I suppose I can write you an order. But honestly, nobody would bother looking into anything else until you were off the Oxycodone."

"So I need to go off now?"

"Oh, yeah. Definitely. But you'll have to wean yourself, because you're going to have withdrawal symptoms if you don't take it slow."

That didn't sound good. "You mean like I'm addicted now?"

"Oh, no no no. You're not *addicted*. You're physically dependent."

"Um…so, what's the difference?"

"Well, obviously you're not going to be an addict, Linda. But your body's gotten used to having this drug. It's going to take some adjusting in your brain to do without it."

"Okay, well then, how do I do it?"

"Oh, you'll need to get your doctor at home to help you with this. Our clinic doesn't do tapering or withdrawal."

That didn't seem right. They prescribe the stuff, but they won't help you get off it?

"It's not like I can just call and get in to see her right away, though. They book weeks ahead. If I'm supposed to get off the drugs, I want to get started. Can't you at least give me a hint?"

He took up a notepad and started sketching out a graph showing how I should cut back five mg each week until I wasn't taking any at all.

"Okay," I said, taking a big breath and letting it out. Apparently that was it then? Just gradually reduce the dose? I folded the paper and stuffed it in my bag. "So when's my next appointment?"

"Oh, five years."

"Really?" In all my less extensive knee surgeries I'd always had several follow-ups.

"Well okay," he said jovially. "Come in at one year if you want to. Come late in the day."

What, like we'd go out and have drinks afterwards?

On one hand, I was pleased to be declared well. But was I? Really?

He was done with me, anyway. I had a new knee. No surgical complications. I'd done my rehab like a good girl. I was a success.

As for this ridiculous dose of Oxycodone I'd been taking—he obviously didn't have to worry about a nice lady like me. Look how motivated I was to get off.

No way would I be the type to become a drug addict.

I started cutting back that very night.

"I'm going off faster than this stupid chart," I told Herb. "Look—by his schedule I won't be completely off until the middle of February. Just that much longer that my brain's used to having this stuff."

"Okay, if you're sure that's what you want to do."

"It is. I want to get off this and then get off the Lexapro and then the Propranolol."

I'd been taking the beta blocker Propranolol for nearly twenty-five years as a migraine preventative. It had reduced the number and severity of my headaches, improved my life and, I'd always joked—probably hoping to beat Herb to it—improved my personality. It kept me from getting so whipped up, thus helping stave off the migraine that inevitably came with the diffusing of a tense situation. But, although my neurologist denied it, I suspected the drug made it hard to keep weight off. After all, I couldn't get my pulse up over a hundred no matter how hard I exercised. Wouldn't that affect my metabolism? Twice previously I'd tried to go off of it, and both times I'd felt like I'd taken speed. Or, at least how I *imagined* speed would feel. My former PCP, Dr. Herrick, dismissed my interest in quitting it and suggested I just be grateful the pharmaceutical companies had developed something that had helped me so much over the years.

But when I'd gone for my last pre-op on my own, my surgeon, Dr. Cramer, said he thought going off Propranolol was a good idea. Something about people shouldn't be going around damped down all the time.

When I'd reported this to Herb, he wasn't enthusiastic.

"Fine for him to say. You go off all this stuff and I'll send you down to go out to lunch with him and see how he likes you then."

Ouch. I understood that change of any kind made my husband uneasy, but seriously? He feared me *not* on drugs?

Now, looking back, it seems odd that Dr. Cramer seemed mildly concerned about my being on Propranolol, but voiced no worries about the Xanax which I had dutifully, repeatedly listed in all the pre-op forms. I will always wonder if he had mixed up the two. At the very least, I now know that concurrent prescriptions for an opioid and a benzodiazepene should have given him pause.

Christmas was lost on us that year. Understand that Herb had been my model for Fun Dad Bill Hummer in my Nekomah Creek books. *Nekomah Creek Christmas* was sparked by his delightful yet maddening enthusiasm for outdoor decorating. In real life, our joke was always that he had to promise to get the dozens of jack-o-lanterns off the porch and out of the orchard trees before he started stringing Christmas lights.

This year, the year from hell, he put up a tree. Period. That was it.

Also, for the first time ever, we agreed to forgo gifts between the two of us. What we needed to give each other couldn't be bought.

Nobody in their right mind would attempt to go full bore on a building project just as they were detoxing, but then, I was *not* in my right mind—I just didn't know it yet. Finishing the Kings Valley cabin was on our To-Do list, simple as that. And as far as my condition, it's not like the surgeon had warned us what lay ahead. I doubt he had any idea. He had declared me well. He wasn't about to be in the business of drug withdrawal any more than he would think to sign on with the cleaning crew swabbing the blood out of the operating room after he'd performed one of his surgeries.

All fall a construction crew had been framing our tiny cabin up in the coast range foothills, a quick half-hour drive from the farm. Now we would undertake the finish work, with me painting and wallpapering while Herb nailed up the wainscoting he and Mary earlier in the fall had laid out on saw horses in the backyard and varnished to a rich amber hue.

As soon as I cut back on the Oxycodone, I felt sick. Dr. Cramer hadn't mentioned anything about this. I went on the internet. Bingo. Nausea was one of the first effects of detox. I started taking the anti-nausea meds he'd given me at my first post-op visit.

I don't look too bad in the pictures of me at this time—they were all taken when my dose had kicked in. Entirely different story when I'd get to the end of the dose and had to tough it out to the next. I felt wretched. Now I not only had pain in my knee, my whole body hurt. Especially distressing was the weird pain in the back of my thighs, *both* thighs. Not exactly an ache, not precisely a burn, it was a creepy, nervy harbinger of the rest of the symptoms coming over me. In bed, I'd have what they call restless leg syndrome, lying there as if I were trying to run somewhere, run away from the drugs.

On cabin work days, I would dose up before climbing into the truck with Herb. By the time we'd opened the gate and driven up the switchback through the old growth, the drugs would be taking effect and I'd be ready to paint. I'd work until I started getting sick again. Then we'd hurry me home to my next pared-down dose and a hot bath. Sometimes we'd drive up separately so that Herb wouldn't have to quit just because I did.

It was during this three-week tapering period that it hit me: this is what it was like to be addicted. And boy, what a lousy way to live. My entire life revolved around the scheduling of the next pill. Except for the brief periods when a dose of Oxycodone was in effect, it was like having a horrid case of the flu. And this is the way it had to be to get clean, I'd read on the internet. If I took enough to *not* feel bad, I was feeding the addiction.

We were in no shape for Christmas.

Bailing us out, Mary and Jaci offered to host the Christmas Eve gathering. A scant hour before we were due at their bungalow near the Oregon State University campus, I was lying in bed, paralyzed with pain.

Kick in. Kick in.

And then the Oxycodone I'd taken on schedule hit my brain. My joints unfroze. I got out of bed, put on my makeup, fixed my hair. I showed up looking perfectly well, I'm confidant, to my kids. But, Cinderella-like, my time was limited. The magic would wear off. I had to scurry home before my gown reverted to rags and my carriage once again became a pumpkin.

My Christmas Day meds were likewise timed. At my mother's house, to the extended family, my brother and his fast-growing clan, I probably looked fine as I, along with everyone else, forked up Herb's popular crab lasagna.

In the days following, I faithfully emailed my mom the progress of my taper, putting the most optimistic spin possible on the whole miserable business. It wouldn't be long now, I assured her, before I was well and able to take her out to lunch. One of her emailed responses opened with this:

Never thought I would get a message from my daughter saying she's going through detox!

Since it was she who'd early on observed to me that people often joke about things they really mean, I couldn't help feeling defensive, and wrote back with more explanations.

Around New Years, she phoned with a cheery *How are you?*

"Awful," I said, the truth popping right out the way it tends to do with me. I'm always forgetting that *How are you?* should not necessarily be answered honestly. "I'm just awful."

"Oh," she said. "Did you get a cold?"

"Mom." I sneezed. Twenty-eight for the day so far. "I'm trying to detox, remember?" I should have been more patient with her 85-year-old memory, I suppose, but my mother was still sharp, and routinely rejected and found insulting any concessions to age.

"Well, I'm sorry," she said, "but I've just never known anybody who had to go through this."

Wait. Was that *shame* I heard? Was there something Freudian in this memory lapse?

In the days ahead I would keep trying to help her understand. I needed her empathy, but I see now I totally underestimated *her* need, which was to believe her daughter's sorry state couldn't possibly have anything to do with drugs.

CHAPTER 7

Having taken the last crumb of Oxycodone on New Year's Eve, I was positively giddy by the time I walked into my appointment with my primary care physician on January 5th. I was more than ready to be a person actually living a life again, and in spite of the trepidation both Herb and I felt at the prospect of my jumping off the narcotic completely, nothing dramatic had happened. Although I felt nauseated, I never actually threw up. I didn't go into seizures or suffer terrible diarrhea.

In acknowledgment of my apparent stability, we'd decided Herb could finally leave me alone long enough to visit his Aunt Catherine in Los Angeles. No, I would not be joining him at the lovely Channel Inn as we'd imagined back in October. Still, a small triumph, that I could finally take care of myself long enough for him to take care of somebody else. After two days away, he'd be returning tonight.

"I'm glad my thyroid test was right on target," I told Dr. Miller, "but the report I got in the mail didn't say anything about the low iron thing. That means it was okay?"

"Well, let's see." She checked the computerized files. "Oh. Well, you *are* a little sub-par."

Great. Wasn't anybody making the connection that if you asked for a test, you'd want to hear about it if the results weren't normal? Dr. Miller wrote the name of an iron supplement on her prescription pad and handed it to me.

"I'm afraid it's expensive."

"I don't care." I'd have happily paid any price for something that might help.

"Now that I'm off Oxycodone," I started explaining, "I've started tapering the Lexapro." I wasn't depressed, I assured her. As soon as I was off that I planned to start tapering the Propranolol.

Dr. Miller glanced at her watch. "So that's what this visit is about? Going off these different drugs?"

I blinked. "Well, yeah." I guess my allotted time was up. Or maybe she needed to know which box to check in labeling my presenting problem. Whatever, I felt uneasy. Didn't my circumstances make me somebody who was supposed to be under medical care?

I walked out and drove straight across town to the vitamin store, stocking up on this recommended elixir.

"I could have started on this stuff four weeks ago," I complained to Herb when he got home that night. "Maybe I'd already be over the fatigue."

"Well, never mind." He hit the internet and started downloading iron-rich recipes.

Lucky me, married to a man enthusiastic over culinary cures. Soon I was eating plates of beans and molasses, big slabs of steak.

Two days later: a miracle. I was sitting in the breakfast nook when I swear, I felt as if a thick fog had lifted off my brain, a cloud I'd been under so long it had become the heavy gray norm. Thank God, I was finally going to be well! This had dragged on so long.

We drove out to check on the cabin. As soon as we had a break in the weather I needed to paint the exterior trim. The forest skyline looked so beautiful, and oh, I was so grateful to finally be emerging from the darkness. I asked Herb to take my picture. I wanted to mark this day—January 10, 2013.

"This," I crowed, "is a first-day-of-the-rest-of-my-life day!"

"Every day is," Herb couldn't resist noting as he snapped the picture, always having found this platitude idiotically obvious.

"Shut up, you know what it means. You know how I feel. Like this is the first day of the rest of my life being *well*."

When I look at that picture now, though, I don't see any real exuberance. I see only my sad innocence.

A day later the plague of symptoms returned. The persistent aching of my lower teeth showed me how this must all be related to my brain's wiring, because what on earth did my teeth have to do with my post-surgery knee? It was so detached, so random.

Herb said it was like a little wizard behind my brain's curtain, trying first one lever, then another. *Let's see if she'll take another pill if I give her that weird pain in the back of her legs. No? What if she just feels too tired to move? That'll bug her!*

He was trying to be encouraging with this metaphor, give me points for not taking more pills. But since for me there was no question of that, I just felt incredibly annoyed that the little brain guy wasn't getting the message: *Can't make me!*

Dragging myself around the loop of my Doug firs one winter afternoon, I was visited by a memory that had haunted me for thirty years. The final knee surgery I'd undergone during that crisis half my life ago had been in Los Angeles, where Herb had taken me in desperation to a famous surgeon who'd been the official doctor for the Rams football team. After the surgery, the doctor had to tell me he couldn't do anything for me; they'd found nothing to fix.

"I'm so sorry for your pain," he said—this big, stooped, white-haired guy. "But I know how hard it is. I'm telling you this as a person who has chronic pain himself. I do believe, though, that it's nothing the human spirit can't overcome."

I was moved by this. I'd heard the *We can't help you* verdict on my knee before, but never delivered with such compassion.

"You have pain too?" I asked him.

He nodded. "It's so bad, sometimes just breathing in air over my teeth hurts terribly."

For three decades I had treasured the memory of his kindness, always remaining haunted by his comment about his teeth. Because—how weird—what kind of chronic pain makes your teeth hurt?

Walking the field that chilly day, my teeth aching, it hit me. I'll bet that poor man was prescribing himself narcotics. God knows he wouldn't be first doctor to do so. Maybe he didn't even understand himself that his pain could have been an inter-dose symptom of tolerance.

January was a blur.

"I'm not getting anything done!" I complained to Herb.

"You're detoxing," he said. "That's not nothing."

So much time in the bathtub, staring morosely at my knee. I hadn't had a good-looking knee in decades; the extension of my original scar from six to eight inches was hardly noteworthy. Still, having to look at it newly purpled was no upper.

Herb systematically rounded up detox supplies. Unfortunately, everything a person could buy to aid somebody in my situation had an inescapably alternative vibe, and Herb is the least woo-woo guy around. Never mind. He sucked it up and lit scented candles wrapped in paper printed with words of affirmation. He downloaded a fresh collection of spa-type music. He bought lotion to give me massages. Seriously, I knew I had it good. I would put the personalized treatment I was receiving here at Wake Robin Farm up against anything the stars were paying big bucks for in Malibu.

In reclaiming this bathroom from the kids when they went off on their own, I'd taken out the shower-tub combo and put in a soaking tub with a subway tile surround. I replaced the cheery, kid-friendly wall paper with a striking reproduction pattern from Bradbury & Bradbury, a gilt enhanced design I'd later seen featured in *American Bungalow*. It was Herb who suggested we go ahead and install grab bars in the tub even though neither of us yet needed them.

"Better to do it before we're trying to scramble around because somebody's going to have surgery or something."

How's that for prescience?

Now, every time I grabbed the bronze finish bars (no need to look institutional) I inwardly—and sometimes out loud—thanked Herb for his foresight.

I was advised to sit in the hot water for a half hour, but I always got too flushed and had to get out, feeling guilty for wasting the Epson salts. I'd wrap myself in a towel and sit on the closed lid of the toilet, my head against the wall, often spending longer trying to summon the energy to rise and get on with it than I had supposedly benefitting from the bath therapy. Sometimes, dizzyingly hot, I'd pull myself up with a grip on the window ledge and crank open the stained-glass panel to let in a puff of foggy winter air.

Eventually, even though I wasn't leaving the house, I'd dress, put on makeup and fix my hair. Part of my Cute Enough to Keep campaign, I told Herb, who always loyally assured me this was not remotely an issue. But to be honest, I was doing it just as much for myself. I'd actually started this when I realized my career would mainly be conducted at home. Other writers gloat about being able to work in their pajamas, but I was always aiming for the psychological boost of self-respect getting dressed might deliver. And now, why pass a mirror and have it depressingly confirmed that while my life had effectively stopped, my aging hadn't? This whole "Health Journey" was no beauty treatment, and I needed all the encouragement camouflage could afford me.

If I wasn't in the bathroom, I could be found in my office, searching the internet for help, advice, comfort—some story that might parallel mine.

This I could never find.

Instead, the message boards regarding opioid addiction and attempts at withdrawal revealed to me an alarming world of hurt out there. Some people were young enough to call in their mothers to care for them, but the middle-aged women….oh, it was heartbreaking. A story of trying to secretly detox while taking care of three small children because if the estranged father found out, he'd take the kids. Women posting about the husbands who were hooked and had lost their jobs and now what the hell were they supposed to do?

No narratives of healing to be found. People posted in the middle of their agonies, seemingly finding solace in detailing their horrific symptoms. Other people posted *Hang in there* messages, but I found no calm voices of experience. Many of the frantic users wanted only to know how soon they had to start detoxing for the job-related drug screening they had coming up. People dishing out advice claimed authority by having been through half-a-dozen detoxes themselves. Great. Nobody ever seemed to get clean for good. The posts were always years old, too, leaving me constantly wondering how these stories had turned out.

I worried these women had become the statistics. An alarming report from the Center for Disease Control stated that opioid overdose deaths had increased five-fold in the decade between 1999 and 2010 among a surprising demographic—middle-aged women. It wasn't hard to understand. A woman's back goes out at work, the doctor gives her pain pills to help. And they do help. They make everything easier. And good Lord, when you have kids, grandkids, husbands, parents, everybody depending on you, what are you going to do? A pill doesn't seem like the worst choice in the world. That little pill gives you a break in the way none of your dependents do.

Sometimes I had trouble picturing the lives of these people. Describing the most dramatic of withdrawal episodes, they would conclude with *And then I almost didn't make it to work.* Really? *Really?* I couldn't see all this throwing up and diarrhea and convulsive shaking coinciding with anything other than lying there being very sick indeed, with work or anything else entirely out of the question.

Still, I kept reading. Perhaps these stories helped maintain my perspective. I didn't have to worry about losing a job. My book royalties (such as they were) would keep coming. I had a loving husband eager to bring home from town anything at all that might ease my pain, speed my recovery. Carrot juice helped detox your liver? He was on it. Ginger beer helped with nausea? Stocking up immediately.

Did it ever actually lessen my agony to have nice wallpaper to stare at? I'll never know. All I can say for sure is that, even being completely conscious of having surroundings as conducive to healing as possible, detox was still a bitch.

Although I'd never actually thrown up, I felt constantly sick to my stomach. One day I staggered into the pharmacy for a refill of my anti-nausea meds.

I liked our pharmacist, Wen, a gentle giant of a Chinese-American who, it turned out, had married a woman whose family, the Changs, had worked on our farm years ago and had become my model for the particularly hard-working Chinese-Cambodian family in my first novel, *Children of the River*. No more farm labor for them these days; Wen's wife, Siv Ching, and most of her siblings had become pharmacists themselves.

"So, when you have to go through withdrawal like this," I asked him now, "how long does it take before you feel better?"

He looked sympathetic. "Two to four weeks."

I groaned. My surgery was four months ago. This was all supposed to be in my rearview mirror by now. Detox was starting to feel like a completely separate recovery.

"It's already been two weeks since I went off the Oxycodone," I told him, signing for the meds.

"Two more weeks, then."

Yeah, I could do the math.

Well, I'd just have to hang in there. Compared to what I'd already been through, two weeks wasn't much.

It's one thing for people to tolerate the regular flu for a week; quite another story to have withdrawal "flu" drag on for weeks or months, all the while knowing if they just took a dose of their opioid med, the symptoms would all go away, even if only temporarily.

I would never again read articles about drug addiction with the same judgmental attitude. In any given addiction narrative of use, abuse, and using again after getting "clean," scant attention is given to the physical consequences of withdrawal. The agony of being so sick. To a reader who's never gone through this, "using" again just sounds like a bafflingly stupid decision. A person would have to be an idiot to go back after detoxing in the first place, right? Movies show the addict twitching on a jail cell floor or twisting in her sheets on a detox facility bed, but there's little recognition that feeling this bad can go on for quite a long time. And these are junkies, right? So a bout of twitching isn't really that horrendous of a punishment, wouldn't you say?

I'm ashamed to admit that's pretty much what I thought. Now it seemed a miracle to me that anyone who didn't have the good fortune of my stable family support ever got and stayed clean. I'm sure I'd been as judgmental as the next person, but for the future, anyone who managed to survive this and not go back to drugs would have my sincerest admiration.

Not that I ever considered taking another Oxycodone tablet myself.

I'm not bragging; I simply knew that reverting to more Oxycodone would be breaking the rules of detox, and as a person with a deep-seated fear of authority, playing by the rules is avoidance behavior on my part. I can't stand to be in trouble.

The bitterest pill for someone like me? Being in trouble precisely because I *did* follow the rules.

In the fifth grade, the fire alarm went off while we were in the locker room, showering after PE. I grabbed a towel and ran outside. That was the rule, right? Just get out fast?

Apparently not. Other girls got dressed. They came out in their own sweet time, while I clutched my towel around my skinny self, all the boys laughing at me. What a ruckus! What hilarity! And to my confounding horror I saw that the teachers were annoyed at *me* for causing it. Apparently I was supposed to somehow know it was just a drill.

Decades later my best friend of that year visited our teacher. She reported to me that when she brought up my name, he gleefully retold the story, saying it was the main thing he remembered about me. Yes, very funny, Mr. Smith—a ten-year-old girl, shivering and mortified. I'm afraid there's not enough tragedy-to-comedy time in my life for this incident to become truly laugh-worthy for me.

But looking back, I realize something crucial about the whole sad business: it continues to anger me in retrospect mainly because this was such poor form on the part of these teachers, who surely shouldn't be in the business of being entertained by a child's humiliating situation. For some other little girl with an ongoing history of abuse, this could have been truly traumatizing.

But as for me—forget it. This would go down as what is referred to as a PTE...a *potentially* traumatic episode. Because I wasn't accepting any shame or guilt. I was just mad. Adults, I saw, could be surprisingly stupid.

I was a little 'fraidy cat. Youngest kid on 34th Street, no way was I letting the big kids ride me on their bicycle handle bars. I implored my mother not to drive on First Street downtown. Too close to the river! We might swerve and dive in! When the big scary cement mixer trucks roared past our little house, I ran in the back yard and shut the picket gate against them.

This business of being a chicken did not extend to social anxiety in any way, though. I couldn't wait to start kindergarten. I clearly remember my four-year-old fantasy: I'd be on the sofa, watching through the picture window as the big kids passed on their way to school. Then one bright, glorious day I'd jump down and fling open the front door. "Wait!" I'd cry, my hand gaily flinging out a greeting. "Wait for me!"

I did have one big fear about starting school. What if I got sick? Then I wouldn't be able to go. I'd be in trouble! No matter how my mother tried to assure me they didn't *want* me to go to school sick, I refused to be mollified. Where did I get this idea? I honestly don't know. In later years I'd be able to cite many instances where my mother modeled sticking-it-out-through-pain behaviors on her own part, or made me feel that having an accident or illness that interrupted fun was rather bad form—we won't get into that—but I remember no such incidents before this start-of-school business. Was something impressed upon me while I was still too young for it to have a chance of becoming part of my conscious memory? Maybe, but since my own three children always seemed to me to have arrived hard-wired with certain distinct traits I could not tie to my particular mothering style, I certainly do not regard it as impossible, the notion that I might simply have been born with this self-imposed guilt trip already in place, the idea that illness always requires a penance.

When my parents bought a slightly bigger house in a new subdivision, it meant I'd have to switch schools in the middle of kindergarten. I could not for the life of me understand why my mother was so concerned how I'd deal with this.

New people? No problem. I was always busier fighting off fears centering on actual physical safety, and I paid serious attention to the rules in this regard.

The one time I exhibited a bit of adventurous defiance came when I was about seven. My parents had cautioned me to steer clear of razor blades, pointing out they were very sharp and could cut and hurt you. One night, lying awake at my ridiculously early bedtime, I decided to put this to my personal test. While my parents were in the living room watching TV, I got up and sneaked across the hall to the bathroom.

Standing on bare tiptoes, I opened the medicine cabinet, drew out one of the forbidden blades and unwrapped it. Then, holding up my left thumb, I carefully drew the sharp edge of the razor across it.

Nothing. My little pink thumb looked just the same. I remember an instant of indignation. *They lied.*

And then the bubbling red line appeared. *Oh, my gosh!*

I remember no pain, only shock. And a certain shame at not having believed my parents. I grabbed a wad of toilet paper to staunch the blood, dashed across the hall and dove back into bed.

Apparently when people warned you about the consequences of certain actions, attention should be paid.

I was the girl in school you hated.

I remember my mother reading me my first grade teacher's comment on my report card: **Linda is very bright, but she doesn't always have patience with other students who don't learn as quickly.**

Yep, that's me. Was I actually supposed to *care*? As long as I wasn't officially in trouble and the gold star Scotch-taped to my desk wouldn't be ceremoniously unpeeled, I wasn't sure I did. I was going to school to learn stuff, after all. Kids goofing off in class were holding me back.

One grownup expression for my brand of impatience is being a person who "doesn't suffer fools gladly," this trait more readily tolerated, lauded even, among males. Bad news for me: I wasn't Steve Jobs; I was female—Little Goody Two-Shoes.

I just couldn't help feeling I could always spot the potential pitfalls in whatever loomed ahead—yes, commonly referred to as being a Know-It-All—and I found it challenging to keep such prescience to myself.

My friend Patty and I used to play in a vacant corner lot with the rest of the neighborhood kids. One day the boys said we could be in their club. Just one admission requirement: we had to pee in front of them.

"Don't do it, Patty," I said. "It's a trick."

But Patty thought it was worth a shot.

It wasn't.

"Ha ha! You did it!" the boys crowed. "You did it!" What a triumph! Funniest thing ever. "Don't you know you can't ever be in our club? You're *girls!*"

I'm sure at eleven I hadn't the good grace to withhold a lofty *I told you so.*

You think Patty found this endearing? Like I said, the girl you loved to hate.

If there's a gene predisposing one to a penchant for risky behavior, I didn't get it. Growing up, I never took a puff of a cigarette, much less a joint. Even though I hung with the drama crowd in high school and everybody else was apparently indulging, I didn't. Didn't drink. Didn't break curfews. I was, in short, NO FUN.

Only once was I naughty with drugs. I was three-and-a-half. I crawled under my baby brother's empty crib with a bottle of children's aspirin and, in the quiet, dusty privacy, enjoyed three or four of the zesty little orange tablets.

My mother found the bottle on the floor and confronted me. Busted! I will never forget her angry alarm.

"I guess a little mouse must have done it," I tried, hoping to assuage her with my light-hearted charm.

Nope. Cute wasn't going to cut it.

All right, all right, I remember thinking. *I won't do it again.* But come on, it was ridiculous how over the top she was acting about this. What, did she think I was stupid? I knew better than to eat the whole bottle.

And how did I know that? Those orange-smelling little aspirins tasted just like candy. Why didn't I just keep crunching them down?

Somebody must have warned me, I'm thinking now. Somebody must have explained to me that medicine wasn't candy.

At sixty-one, I was still that same little girl, fully capable of absorbing useful information and understanding consequences.

I wish somebody had taken the trouble to explain to me about Oxycodone and how it works.

Explained *before* I got addicted.

I'd been carefully counting off the days to the four weeks the pharmacist predicted would be the outer limit of this awful withdrawal process.

At twenty-eight days, I felt no better. I felt tricked. I felt like I'd peed in front of the boys and they still wouldn't let me into their club.

I wrote an impassioned letter to my surgeon. He should know, I thought, for the sake of his future patients, just how far short of glowing the outcome of this "highly motivated patient" had been. I'd done everything according to direction and yet here I was, dope sick as any recovering addict who'd been snorting this stuff recreationally for years. I told him I'd found stories on the internet that made me wonder if the Lexapro I'd been on had actually been blocking the pain relieving effects of the narcotics. Could that be why I'd found myself needing such high doses just to stay out of torturous pain? Doctors shy from anecdotal evidence, but when a recreational drug user asks on-line what's up with the fact that he can't seem to get high on his usual Oxys now that he's on Lexapro and somebody else writes back, **Dude, save your money. Everybody knows you can't get high from that if you're on Lexapro….**Well, hey, I'm sorry— that has more ring of truth to me than anything posted by a given drug's own manufacturer.

I have never sued anybody, I wrote the surgeon, **and if I ever get my life back, the last thing I'd want to be doing is spending time in court haggling over money. However, I do feel I've been subjected to unnecessary pain and suffering, and I'm writing this**

in hopes it will help you improve your health care delivery so that future patients will not have to go through this.

I do wish I had been better informed about the way narcotics work on the brain. If I'd known then what I know now, that the opiates actually sensitize you to pain, and that the pain I'd feel on cutting back the dosage was not so much post-surgery pain as it was the drugs screaming for me to take more, I would have started much sooner to fight this monkey off my back.

CHAPTER 8

The cabin in Kings Valley had been a bone of contention from the start. We didn't even want to build it. The county said we had to, though, if we wanted to preserve the *right* to build. This is why you see a lot of ugly little white trailer houses on Oregon tree farms—an unintended consequence of Oregon's tight land use laws, which in general, of course, we support. So, although we had no plans ourselves for ever building a big log McMansion on this 155-acre forest parcel we had acquired from Weyerhaueser, we had to build a minimal structure, and no, a cute little "tiny house" on wheels like you see on HGTV wouldn't cut it as permanent in Benton County.

At four hundred and twenty square feet, it's quite possible the planning and construction of our little cabin may have broken some kind of record for a building project yielding the most hours of arguing per square foot. But finally it was turning out quite satisfactorily.

To our surprise and delight, we discovered that while the Willamette Valley was socked in with a layer of pea-soup fog, our forest property lay just above it. Driving the last rise of the Kings Valley Highway felt like swimming up out of a murky pool and bursting into the light. Sunlight was supposed to be good for me, and I loved sitting on that porch, relishing the way the orientation Herb had asked me to designate for the cabin had worked out so well. Nice feng shui!

The porch ran the entire width of the cabin, and I had always maintained that the broad steps should too. Maybe I was remembering the log cabin craft house on the lakeshore at Camp Kilowan, where I'd gone as a girl. But Herb wanted steps narrower and less expensive. In the meantime, one of the carpenters had mistakenly knocked up a set which were as narrow as Herb wanted, but too steep. They had to be redone anyway.

The two of us were sitting there one day taking a break, soaking in the sun. The green exterior trim had gone on quite nicely for me, and Herb seemed satisfied with the way the project had turned out, even if he did leave it to other visitors to rave about the clever cuteness of it all.

"When you see how this place is really all about this porch facing west," I ventured, "you can see why I'd still like to have the steps running all the way across the front, right?" I was so enjoying this warm little moment of returning confidence in myself.

"No, I don't," he said, "and I thought we already settled this."

Uh-oh. I took a breath. I'd grown accustomed to soft, careful conversations.

"But since they have to re-do the steps, isn't it still up for debate? And now you don't have to try picturing it from sketches. You can sit here and just *see* it would be better."

"Wide steps still cost more. That was the point. Not just what you thought would be nice."

"Not that much more in the scheme of the whole thing, though. And if that's what really makes the cabin...."

"So where does it stop with you? No expenses spared? Just spend any amount on this place?"

What was he talking about? Every decision we'd made had taken cost into account. The cabin wasn't my idea. All I'd done was figure out how to make something attractive and appropriate out of our compliance with the laws. Did he really regret we weren't crouching on the narrow stoop of an eye-sore white trailer house right about now?

"I'll pay for the wider steps out of my writing money," I offered. I kept a separate account just for the pleasure of tracking what I'd earned on my own. I liked spending the money on projects I particularly wanted to promote, the ones where Herb was dragging his feet. Putting my money where my mouth was, as I thought of it.

"Where the money comes from doesn't matter," Herb said.

Okay, you win, I thought, feeling myself crumpling inside. *I won't care about the steps. Actually, I don't.* He hadn't barked at me like this since before the surgery. He was probably entitled to be worn out always trying to nice to me, but didn't he get what a big deal managing to actually feel engaged about *anything* was for me? My grasp was so tentative. I was dangling from a high ledge. I hardly needed him stomping on my fingers. I was perfectly capable of letting go all on my own.

I stared dully at the ridgetop horizon, dragged down by a painful insight. My husband liked me better sick than well. With me weak and weepily grateful for his tender sickbed ministrations, he could feel like a hero. The first little hint of the real me coming back, the *old* me, energetic and bossy—well, that wife just seemed to annoy the hell out of him.

From that point on, every time I went on another of the heavy emotional downers that proved part of the withdrawal process, I'd have trouble accepting my husband's kindnesses without a twinge of suspicion. The horrid little voice in my brain that sounded exactly like mine was all too quick with the insidious whispering: *Don't trust this guy! Look at him, acting all sweet. Haven't you noticed he's the one who's right there ready to smack you back down the minute you feel the least bit better?*

He'd been my loving caregiver; now I felt a shift to something new. He had become my keeper.

My mother finally persuaded me to go out to lunch, her sure-fire prescription for any less-than-sunny mood.

"So, how are you?" she asked across the table at Big River downtown.

I hesitated. "The thing is, I'll get better for a little while, but before I can even write people and say I'm well, all the symptoms come back. It's just incredibly frustrating."

"But you feel better right now?"

"Um, yeah." I picked at my crab cake. "Right this minute I'm not too bad."

"Okay, so you're better, then."

It wasn't a question. It was a firm indicator we needed to move on to some fresh topic. Enough, already, with the tedious recitation of my malingering. My mother's a survivor of deadly accidents and a firm believer in the power of positive thinking. She'd want to see me simply ignore whatever symptoms were still plaguing me and get on with it.

Besides, in her book, people had surgeries and they recovered; she had. Her summation of the whole issue the last time we'd spoken on the phone was this: "Well! I'll bet you'd never go and take drugs like this again, would you?"

You naughty little girl! Let's just hope you learned your lesson!"

That's how it sounded to me, anyway.

Still, pathetically, I'd tried to defend myself, saying I most probably *would* take narcotics again if I ever found myself in that degree of unbearable pain. I tried to explain how I felt tricked, how the doctors hadn't explained about withdrawal pain blah blah blah. Wow. I even bored myself.

Encounters like this were ever more frequently making me want to take Xanax. Up until now, I'd used it almost entirely as a sleep aid, especially when I was on the brain-busying Oxycodone. But now I found myself reaching for that plastic bottle in the middle of the day. I just couldn't cope. And apparently people in opioid withdrawal were prescribed benzodiazepines (Xanax, Valium, Ativan etc.) to help them through it. Didn't I have every reason to be anxious? I just couldn't seem to get well. The fact that other people seemed to be thinking I ought to just made the whole thing worse.

As I began confiding my situation to a few people, other real-life painkiller stories started coming back to me. One gym buddy's husband had broken his clavicle in a bicycle accident. Coming off the necessary narcotics, he'd been slammed with a depression so profound, he hardly knew what hit him. When I visited him as my friend requested, he told me he'd never had any prior tendency toward depression, and now regretted his lack of empathy and understanding for those who had.

Another woman's thirty-something son had been on pain meds for a bad back. He was promising to go off, he said, but first had to deal with the toothache that was plaguing him. I should have explained to her about toothache being a common inter-dose withdrawal symptom, I thought later, but it wouldn't have mattered. He wasn't about to quit. Still hooked, last I heard.

Another acquaintance confided that her son had been in a car accident at eighteen, walked out with a big bottle of Oxycodone and, three years later, hasn't been the same since. "Completely unproductive" was her expression. She suspects he's moved on to street drugs.

Nobody ever had a story of comfort, of healing after long-term use.

"Sounds like you need a support group," another gym buddy said.

Right, but where were they?

I could just see myself at Narcotics Anonymous or some such group meeting where everybody's supposed to support each other to not "use" again. I doubt anyone would appreciate my pointing out I'd only ever followed my doctor's orders. And what would they make of my insistence I had no cravings? All I could see was one more round of being the girl they'd love to hate.

CHAPTER 9

"Time to start trying for a baby," Miles announced across the restaurant table where we'd taken him and Ziwei for a Chinese New Year celebration dinner in late February. He made a crack about holding off on a bottle of a certain drink brother Will had given him, one that contained a substance known to diminish the quality of a man's sperm. "I'll save it to celebrate. Shouldn't be long."

My eyes widened at Herb. Our son's bravado! What if they had trouble conceiving? I couldn't picture Miles staying as calm as his father had—not if, like us, they ended up needing cycle after cycle of treatment for infertility.

I was shocked, too, at Miles being so blunt with his revelation. Like most of my friends, I was eager for grandchildren, but I'd been trying to school myself to simply await and celebrate the thrilling news of a pregnancy whenever our kids chose to deliver it.

Now that he'd put the idea in my head, though, there'd be no taking it back.

My mind turned straight to houses, and the fact that they might soon be needing a bigger one. Stealth House Hunting became my therapy during this time, the only thing that seemed to distract me from how bad I was feeling.

I've always wondered if my love of house hunting is a result of actually having had so little chance to do much of it as we were starting out.

When I was trying to convince Herb we should get married, I asked my mother why she thought he was stalling. He clearly wanted to be with me, and I'd made it clear I wasn't moving in with him unless we were married, not with my parents and grandparents living right here in Corvallis. Nobody would have batted an eye about this just a few years later, but unmarried co-habitation wasn't going to fly in 1973, not with Herb teaching middle school. Besides, I could see how hard it was for this guy to accept change. If I moved in with him and everything was just as he wanted it, I'd be begging for commitment forever.

"He needs a house," my mom said. "Maybe you should help him find one."

So, for the very first time in my life, I called a Realtor. The first place Herb looked at sold before I could get away from my job at the flower shop to go look at it. The second, a ramshackle farm way out in the coast range, was inaccessible due to flooding on the Marys River. The third—this is a fairytale, remember—was a circa 1917 house on Wake Robin Lane.

The Realtor took us to see it. Herb instantly fell in love with the setting—country acreage on the Marys River at the end of a quiet road. Yes, he'd been saying he wanted to live beyond the noise of town and, standing in the gravel driveway, we could definitely hear the dull, distant hum of traffic. But, so what? You *felt* like you were way out in the country, and mature oak trees were not something you could have in your lifetime if you had to start them from acorns.

The structure itself had never been more than the humblest of farmhouses, but it had the wide front porch we'd dreamed of, and I could already see that a dormer room on the front (in which I'm now writing these words) would break up that steep roof and give the place a balanced craftsman look. As Herb inspected everything, I followed him around. Wake Robin Farm (how cool was it that the street had been named after this place?) had been a chicken ranch, and every rusting piece of caging and equipment was still lying around. Trash officially dealt with had been thrown over the side of the dip into the lower floodplain meadow just outside the kitchen window. At the bottom lay a rusted-out car. My first project would definitely be calling in a giant trash bin.

The house didn't have the fireplace I'd always wanted. Or even a shower. The kitchen/bathroom wing had been haphazardly tacked on sometime after initial construction. That whole section would have to go. The asking price was suspiciously low; the tax assessor's valuation disturbingly so. Face it—the place was a dump.

But following my handsome true love around the place, I merely murmured approval. If he bought this place, it meant we were getting married. That's all that mattered to me.

I'll never forget poking my head out the door at Kessey's Flowers, looking up Monroe Avenue to see Herb's wooden-bumpered VW van parked at the Benton County Courthouse. He was doing official papers! He was buying Wake Robin Farm!

I would not be long at Kessey's. I had better things to do than drive a van of funeral flowers to the cemetery for $1.60 an hour. Especially in the short skirt and panyhose my log-truck-driving, flower-shop-owning boss insisted I wear no matter how bitter the cold. No, not even that recent five-cent raise above minimum wage could dissuade me (!)

I had better plans. I was going to marry my own true love, put on overalls, and get busy on the project of a lifetime.

We've always marveled how our young naivety and impulsiveness had resulted in a home we've been satisfied with ever since.

Okay, wait. Let's not be disingenuous. It's not that tidy. More accurately, we've been satisfied with the *location*. And full disclosure: if we hadn't had the dumb luck of Herb's badass great-grandmother leaving bits of money to every descendent with the good sense to get themselves born before she died (Herb squeaked in) so that we'd be able to fix our idiot oversights—*You kids never notice this house got no foundation? Your septic system just a crappy ole rusted-out tank?*— we'd have been sunk.

Actual happiness with the house itself lay many remodeling projects down the road.

One scene of major dissatisfaction early on involved me in the tub when a mouse skittered through the bathroom. My sustained shriek sent the critter back to the hole under the hot water heater and brought Herb barreling down the insanely steep stairs that ended, inelegantly, at the bathroom door. I had leapt to the edge of the tub. Herb charged in, throwing his arms around my middle, insisting I get down before I fell, but nothing doing, not with a mouse running around.

(I'm thinking now this might have made the funniest, most visibly appealing reality TV show scene of our marriage—both of us stark naked, still young, slender and unscarred by my upcoming C-sections and Herb's eventual emergency splenectomy.)

The tone of my hollering ratcheted up from alarm to anger when it became apparent that this mouse was no stranger to Herb, nor was his entry hole. Apparently I had just married a guy who would not be inclined to nail the necessary flattened can over such a hole until a moment of drama such as this made it mandatory.

But I digress. The point is: for better or for worse, our swift decisiveness and never-look-back commitment to Wake Robin Farm hadn't made for a particularly entertaining search. And now, forty years later, the possibility of a grandchild was just the excuse I needed to happily take up the diversion of playing House Hunters.

I started scouting a pretty new neighborhood not far from our farm, but while biking around the riverfront paths at Willamette Landing seemed to perk me up, it annoyed Herb no end.

"What if she can't get pregnant? Think how sad it would be if we helped set them up in a big house and then they don't have any children to fill it."

"Just because we had trouble doesn't mean they will. But, okay. I promise I won't say anything about it until they're pregnant."

"We aren't even in a position to help them."

"But we'll be selling Jackson Avenue," I reminded him. The bungalow in which they were now living was one of my projects, and they were renting it from us. "They'll be moving into a *lower*-priced house. I could argue they're currently living in more house than they can afford and we're subsidizing them. Besides, I would really like to stop being everybody's landlord."

This probably made too much sense; it took Herb a minute to lob another argument.

"You don't even know what kind of a house they'd want."

"Um, excuse me? You're the one who says I'm not allowed to talk to them about it."

But never mind. I knew I could find a house they'd like.

I emailed my Realtor friend, Clare Staton, for the scoop on Willamette Landing.

Clare and I go way back. At seventeen, I was her counselor at Camp Kilowan. I can still picture her at twelve—already lovely, already towering over me, with clear, pale green eyes and a long dark braid down her back. Fast forward and she was Miles's kindergarten teacher. Her kids and mine later befriended each other in school. See what can happen if you stick around in the same town all your life?

Because she'd eventually quit teaching and become a Realtor, it was naturally Clare I called when, in the winter of 2008, I got the brilliant idea to take a look at the little bungalow on Jackson Avenue. I had always admired it, and now this neglected charmer had been on the market for months. It needed me. And our newly-married kids needed a better-located place to live than their apartment on the far side of town. Here, if Ziwei got a job at Presbyterian Pre-school—the very daycare Miles had attended at the age of three—she'd have a one-block walk to work. And Miles would love being only a half-block from the library. Somehow I just knew if I didn't get to be the one to choose the colors for that house and oversee the transformation, I was going to regret it. And regret is something I strongly believe in avoiding.

I enlisted Clare to show it to Herb with me on Valentine's Day. The owner and I dickered off and on for a few months and, by May, I was tearing the ivy off the ugly chain-link fence that ran between the bungalow and the bigger house on the corner. I spent the whole summer on the project, coordinating contractors and painting the interior, and by September it was ready for Miles and Ziwei. The location had worked out nicely for them, especially with Ziwei getting that job at Presbyterian Pre-school I'd envisioned. But with Miles needing a home office, a two-bedroom house with no bathtub was immediately going to be too small if they had a baby. Especially if the baby's other set of grandparents came to visit from China.

Willamette Landing was growing in popularity, Clare told me, teeming with young families, just the sort I was hoping Miles and Ziwei would very soon become.

"You're completely jumping the gun!" Herb would protest every time I went to yet another open house out there. "You don't even know if she can get pregnant."

"True, but what's the harm in...*informing* ourselves about the neighborhood?"

I was just trying to stay a step ahead. Besides, I was a person whose brain's reward system had been loused up. That's how withdrawal works: accustomed to the artificial opioids of Oxycodone, your own brain ceases its efficient production of dopamine, critical for energy and motivation. It's difficult to take pleasure in anything. People talk about being hooked on *Angry Birds* or *Candy Crush*, or having trouble stopping themselves from playing just one more game of on-line solitaire. I've never been into any of that, but I'm sure if I were sitting at the computer scanning real estate listings with my brain hooked to one of those imaging machines, all the little pleasure areas would be glowing. So, naturally, despite Herb's disapproval, I kept at it.

At least the addictive properties of house hunting didn't come in the form of a pill.

As soon as I'd finished with Oxycodone, I started my quick, two-week taper off of Lexapro. The first time I went weepy over some sentimental TV commercial I thought, *Hey, check it out. I'm not on Lexapro anymore.* And maybe Herb couldn't tell the difference in bed, but I could.

Now for the Propranolol. First seven weeks—no trouble. No speedy feeling. But during the final days at a quarter of my original dose, I was hit with a sinus headache. The first day I took no Propranolol at all it slammed me full force: the aggravating pain that would dog me for eight months to come, biting every afternoon around three o'clock.

Since I'd been taking this beta-blocker all these years as a migraine preventative, my first thought was to grab my migraine meds. But, nothing doing, Imitrex didn't touch this.

Sharp pain stabbed like a red hot spike driven into my left sinus cavity. My teeth on that side ached so bad I'd have run for a dental x-ray except for remembering a milder version of a headache like this I'd had a few years previously when I'd done just that and the x-ray had been clear.

Once more I turned to the internet, searching for symptoms relevant to opioid withdrawal. Bingo. Hyperalgesia. Whatever's going to hurt, hurts worse. I'd always had a tendency toward sinus problems. A cold for me could easily become a sinus infection. Maybe the opioid withdrawal symptoms were taking aim at my own personal Achilles heel.

But the pain! This was ridiculous. I was taking the maximum dose of Tylenol allowed and it was still excruciating, worse than any migraine I'd ever had and I'd had hundreds. That night I stood over a steaming saucepan, frantically dipping in a washcloth and pressing it to my cheek.

"I can't stand it!" I screamed to Herb.

"So, what is it on the scale?" he said, now fully conversant in the med-speak of pain.

"Ten! If I'm screaming, it's a ten!" I went in and threw myself on the bed with the heating pad over my face. "Call somebody," I begged him.

"Like a doctor?"

"Yeah! Like somebody who can tell us what to do! What can I take?"

Pain itself can't actually kill you, right? You probably pass out first anyway. I flashed on stories of people having themselves hauled to the emergency room in the grip of a frightening headache. I'd never done that for a migraine, but this felt bad enough I briefly considered it. But wait. No. Some well-meaning intern would probably shoot me up with narcotics and I'd have to go back to square one on the withdrawals. I hadn't suffered through three months of this crap to start over.

Oh, God, gimme a break. While Herb made a call I lay there, eyes shut tight against the pain, against the darkness of the universe that seemed to press down on me through the bedroom ceiling. What had I done to deserve this? I thought of the big plastic bottle of Oxycodone stashed behind the towels. One tab and this would stop. But then I'd be starting detox all over again. If I was going to take Oxycodone, I probably ought to just go ahead and take enough to finish myself off. But no, I could see how that would go. I'd be in the hospital having my stomach pumped and *then* be back at square one. I did not want to be dead. I just wanted to be out of pain.

"I got a guy," Herb said, finally coming back in. "He says acetaminophen is processed by your liver and ibuprofen by your kidneys, so you can actually alternate and take the max of both without hurting yourself."

"Did you tell him I'm in opioid withdrawal?"

"I didn't see any point in getting into that."

"Oh, for God's sake! Why not? Isn't that the headline here?"

The next morning, we showed up at the opening of Immediate Care along with all the other poor souls who, due to their own illnesses, had just endured horrible Saturday nights.

I told my story, and the doctor confirmed the protocol of using the two different OTC pain meds. He prescribed antibiotics, in case it was a sinus infection. Having had plenty of these in the past, I felt confident it wasn't. Still, I'd take anything that might help without undoing the progress I'd made in withdrawing from Oxycodone.

"And I shouldn't even think of taking any more Oxycodone, right? Even though one little crumb would make the pain go away?"

What a stupid thing to say. I knew the answer. Maybe I was fishing for some credit. Encouragement.

"No, you wouldn't want to be waking up those receptors." And then, with sudden, fresh interest: "You don't have any of that still lying around, do you?"

"Well, my surgeon gave me enough to take forever tapering off. I wanted to get off quicker, so, yeah, I had a lot left."

"Okay, you get rid of that."

I straightened my shoulders defensively. "I'm not going to *take* it."

"Yeah, well, like I said, you get rid of it." He scribbled something on his pad.

I looked at Herb, gave a shrug. "Okay."

But in the parking lot, I told Herb I wasn't so sure. Initially, he'd been the one to suggest hanging on to the remaining pills. Not surprising; he was the one who always had to go through so much trouble to get them.

"We paid for them," he'd said. "We might need them some day."

Fine by me. I was picturing some end-of-the world scenario, somebody's leg pinned under a fallen beam after that massive earthquake that's supposedly going to "make toast of everything west of I-5," according to an article in The New Yorker.

"But maybe keeping them makes me feel strong," I said now. "I can say 'Look, I have them right here and I'm not taking any.'"

"So keep 'em," Herb said, "if it makes you feel better."

"Okay, whatever." I got in the car and fastened my seatbelt. "But don't you love how that doctor seems to feel he's done his job if he states for the record he's advising me not to take narcotics anymore? So he's covered himself. Great. I wish somebody would actually *help* me."

My friend Lynne was the only person I knew who understood the difficulties of trying to live a life while in drug withdrawal. She swore by the acupuncture treatments that helped her through her long taper and recovery from a disastrous month of prescribed Klonopin, and at her recommendation, I booked a young Chinese-American woman.

Rose Tian was about my daughter-in-law Ziwei's age, with a pleasing round face and black hair cut in a simple bob. Since Ziwei's parents are both artists and their work graces our walls, I felt right at home to hear that the beautiful paintings in Rose Tian's office were the work of *her* mother. I loved the haunting Chinese music she played too. I'd listened to a similar playlist the entire time I worked on my memoir about our trip to China for Miles's and Ziwei's wedding.

Rose Tian sat me in a chair, felt my pulse, invited me to begin.

I started spinning out my tortuous tale, hardly pausing for breath. The older you get, the more you've lived through, the longer it takes to give a comprehensive medical history. Tedious, the way it just keeps adding up. I emphasized the recent surgery and drug withdrawal, resorting to flashbacks for the story of my much operated-upon knee. I was wound up, rattling off the pertinent facts as efficiently as possible, aware of the time constraints under which these medical professionals usually seem to be laboring.

But as I talked, Rose Tian listened patiently, her sweet face sympathetic. She did not look at her watch or her notes. Her eyes remained on mine and she let me talk until she was absolutely sure I was finished.

And then she uttered three sentences that struck me as profound: "You are doing everything right. And you are going to get well. But you have to stop trying so hard."

Wow. She took my breath away. She'd nailed it. She'd nailed *me*. I was so Type A. So American. I wanted to be well and I wanted it *now*. Maybe I just needed to be more Asian, more Zen about the whole thing. Yes, surely this was the key.

So I climbed up on the table and let her insert the needles here and there. She would get my *chi* going again. I relaxed. I was going to get well now. All I had to do was stop trying so hard.

CHAPTER 10

Think of others.

Anyone who's ever flipped through a women's magazine or sat through a church service knows this is the standard prescription for whiny self-absorption.

But—think of others? I couldn't. Not in withdrawal. I was completely preoccupied with the physical and mental misery I simply could not ignore. And even if, in a flashing moment of wellness, I hit on an idea of something I might do for or with someone, I couldn't commit to it. Not when I never knew if I'd be well enough, when the time came, to keep my promise.

Lynne said her method had been to say, simply, "I'll be there if I can." Okay, fine, if you're talking about group gatherings and nobody's counting on you personally, but you couldn't just not show up for a lunch date. You couldn't say "Maybe" if you were asked to give a slide talk to a class reading one of your books. What if you woke up that day flattened by a wave of withdrawal? You'd have to call and cancel, ruining people's plans, painfully aware you probably sounded like the worst sort of flake.

Maybe I was being punished. Maybe this was my comeuppance. Because I was the very sort of person who, before I found my own formerly organized self in this position, would have been suspiciously judgmental of a person forever cancelling over mysterious and vaguely explained illnesses.

One commitment I did manage to keep was chauffeuring my non-driving friend Eleanor to the funeral of the father of our mutual friend, Nancy.

"Well, look at you!" Nancy said at the reception afterwards.

What. I glanced over my shoulder. Did she mean me?

"The way you're walking around."

Oh, right. That. People were probably thinking I was a no-show all this time because of my knee. They didn't get that it was all about my brain. But it was spring by now. My September surgery was almost seven months ago—ancient history. I'd forgotten about being a post-knee-replacement-surgery patient; I was busy being a recovering drug addict.

Lynne was also at the reception, and the relief of running into my withdrawal confidante unleashed me. Holding my cup of punch and plate of cheese and crackers, I'm afraid I began ranting in a quiet, but intense and frankly alarming fashion. Since I was the driver, I hadn't damped myself down with the Xanax I might have otherwise, so she was getting a full-force delivery. And before, I'd only discussed this with her privately; now her poor husband was having to hear it. Sorry, Jeff. I could see that glaze going over his eyes, that pulling back.

I watched myself. I heard the desperation in my voice. I probably sounded like an escaped asylum patient who had a couple of uniformed guys looking for me out in the church vestibule, first responders hoping to lead me gently away without the use of restraints.

Maybe this is when I started turning genuinely anti-social. Not agoraphobic. I had no morbid fear of open, public places. I had no problem leaving the house or being around strangers. It was the people I knew I no longer cared to see.

The old me delighted in my inability to execute a list of errands around town without budgeting an extra hour for visiting with people I'd meet down on tree-lined Second Street or in Grass Roots Bookstore. Newly moved here from San Francisco, Eleanor would join my strolls and keep bursting out in laughter. "I don't believe it! You know everybody!"

But now I didn't care to show the people I knew the person I'd become.

I know, I know. Picture me waving off in annoyance your immediate suggestion, that a person needn't be bleeding out her medical details in every casual conversation in the first place.

This seemed different. Completely preoccupied by my strange and ongoing illness, I failed utterly at faking cheerfulness. I was so *not* fine.

"Well, I'm okay as far as the surgery," I'd tend to start out when people asked about it, "but I've been having trouble getting off the drugs."

Mistake. People would draw back. *Trouble with drugs.* How much was I still taking? Then I'd be backpedaling, trying to explain, feeling defensive. *No, see, this is how wicked this stuff is, how bad it messes you up even after you've stopped taking it.* I read in their eyes polite suspicion.

Still, against my better judgment, part of me couldn't help telling this story of addiction and withdrawal as a cautionary tale. *Hey people, this is happening to a lot of people out there. If it could happen to me, it could happen to anyone, so if you have to take painkillers, be sure to get off as quick as you can.....*

I must have seemed slightly demented. Weirdly evangelical. Lacking all dignity. I was telling stories that would make people instantly want to hear the whole thing from some other calmer, saner-sounding point of view.

Have you run into Linda Crew lately? She's acting so strange.

It became easier to just stay home. I hadn't been to church since before the surgery and, funny thing, week after week, I just didn't feel like going back. Not much of a joiner in the first place, it wasn't like I had to cancel a roster of group activities. I simply became the recluse of Wake Robin Farm.

Too bad Emily Dickinson's dead. We could have set up a private support group.

A birthday party for me? Forget it. What's to celebrate? The cold April rain perfectly matched my grim mood. Herb would gladly have mounted a family dinner, but I wasn't up to the assumed but unnoticed pre- and post-cleaning this would require of me. Figured instead I'd just try to drive to Lowe's in Eugene and pick up a batch of light fixtures I'd ordered. Maybe crossing this one thing off my To-Do list would make me feel better.

In the Lowe's lighting aisle, I immediately realized one of the pendants I'd ordered based on an internet picture was too big. I craned up at my replacement choices, wincing at the cavernous store's fluorescent lights. Do they actually buzz or was this just my tinnitus? My teeth ached and the backs of my thighs burned with that creepy nerve pain. If I didn't know this was withdrawal and not the flu, I'd have never gotten out of bed this morning. Honestly, this one simple errand should not have felt like such an overwhelming challenge.

I fished for my cell to ask Will for the ceiling height measurement in his stairwell again.

Like a lot of other University of Portland parents, we had invested in a neighborhood house where Will could live and serve as junior landlord to his buddies, always with the idea that when it came time to sell, I would enjoy the project of fixing the place up, staging it as the lovely family home it could surely be. Long since having graduated, Will was now moving to Bend, his lofty goal to park himself as close to his beloved Mt. Bachelor as possible, see how many days in the snowy season he could make it up there, how many vertical feet he could tally having skied down.

These light fixtures were part of my agenda for the Animal House spiff up.

"So, Mom," Will said, betraying not the slightest impatience at having to take the measurements for me again, "you'll be glad to know that for your birthday gift I decided I *wouldn't* go up skiing at Hood today. I knew you'd probably hear that the roads were bad and you'd be worried about me."

"Oh." That was my birthday gift? "Well, actually I hadn't heard, but it's always nice to *not* have something to worry about, I guess."

Maybe we'd almost done too good of a job, I remember thinking, of convincing these kids of ours that nothing in the world was ever more important to us than them.

Back home, though, I walked in to find the beautiful flower arrangement he'd sent.

I picked up the phone. "You little joker! Good job, honey. They're perfect."

Will laughed, delighted to have played me so effectively.

I loved that he knew me so well. I loved that he'd come through. I've always told my sons they could never go wrong sending flowers to a woman of any age, and I was tickled with this evidence he'd been paying attention.

Miles and Ziwei paid me a birthday visit later that day. I was eager to tell them all about the Chinese acupuncturist.

"She was amazing," I said. "She listened to my whole story and then she said, 'You're doing all the right things.'" And here I leaned forward to emphasize the import. "*But you have to stop trying so hard.*'" I waited, looking from one to the other for affirmation.

"Oh, come on, Mom," Miles said. "She tells you to chill and you think that's so amazingly wise?" The corners of his mouth went dramatically down. "You're smarter than that, aren't you?"

Tears sprang to my eyes. He might as well have smacked me, the way the pain in my left sinus zinged. Was I stupid, finding a little crumb of hope in what had sounded to me—yes, I wasn't ashamed of it—like wisdom? Rose Tian had made me feel a little better, she'd given me hope, and now he had to rip that away? I started to cry. I looked at Herb. Wasn't he going to stick up for me?

Nope. Never had in the past. Wasn't going to start now.

Put a lid on it, Miles. That's all he had to say. That would have helped.

Similar scenes had been enacted by our cast of characters many times in the past, and no doubt would be in the future. I was used to having to defend myself. But right now I just couldn't. I felt too fragile. All I could do in reaction was crumple and cry.

Afterwards Herb pointed out I ought to know Miles was hardly the last word on what constituted wisdom and what didn't.

Yeah, so what? That wasn't the point.

Lucky I didn't know then that this sort of thing was going to get a whole lot worse before it got better.

Or maybe I should say, before *I* got better.

I managed a birthday lunch with Mary the next day, but in order to keep from crying in the restaurant, I had to drug myself with Xanax beforehand. At least with my daughter, though, I knew I wouldn't have to be "on."

This was not the case with my mother. I could not be cheerful enough to suit her, and had to cancel the lunch we'd booked the day following.

This was terribly sad. For both of us. My mother and I had enjoyed a best-friend sort of relationship ever since I'd emerged from adolescence and gone off to college. She wanted to see me get well. She would have loved to count herself part of the solution to my baffling problem. But her protocol of absolutely insisting on fun, and the sunny charm that had cheered her family members and legions of friends through various bouts of gloom over the years simply wasn't going to work on me now.

I didn't feel safe with her. Besides, if wellness could have been conjured by a demand for positive thinking, I would have long ago demanded it of myself.

When I wrote to my surgeon at the end of January, I did not expect to ever hear from him, so when I finally did, it took me by surprise. He wrote that he had initially been "somewhat taken aback" by my letter. He had subsequently re-read it several times, he said, and based on my comments, had begun scheduling his first post-op appointments sooner than the six weeks which had been the clinic's protocol. Although he used the words "sorry" and "apologize" in the carefully passive way that people who parse these things will point out does not come across as satisfactory, I imagine he was sticking his neck out with his legal department to be using these words at all, no matter how they were framed.

He had knocked his lights out searching for studies showing Lexapro blocked the effects of Oxycodone. It seemed to me he wanted to make sure he hadn't blown some cookbook-medicine type directive: If a patient is taking A, do not give her B. The sort of thing that might make him squirm on the witness stand if I took him to court. Well, no worries, Doc. The evidence was all safely anecdotal, which is to say easily, routinely dismissed by the medical community, never mind that it's usually the anecdotes of patients, the stories they tell of the effects of any given drug, that lead to important discoveries of horrific side effects. Don't be counting on the pharmaceutical companies to pay for studies revealing the negative outcomes involving their products.

His only mention of the Oxycodone, the headline of my story as far as I was concerned, was this:

I assure you my intention was not to cause you to become dependent on narcotic medication. [Good to know!] **I gave you a prescription at your follow up visit simply because of your concern about the amount of pain you were experiencing.**

Simply? *Simply?* Nothing about the administration of opioid painkillers is simple, and believing it is can have terrible consequences.

And I had been "concerned" about my pain? No, I beg your pardon—I'd been *concerned* about the heavy dose of narcotics I was having to swallow to damp it down to tolerable levels. And he'd done nothing but assure me I needn't worry.

This man is probably one of the nicest, most personable doctors out there. But nice hadn't helped me. Nice probably isn't helping a lot of other patients when their doctors put being agreeable ahead of their patients' long-term best interests.

Patients need their pain to be acknowledged, not dismissed. They need sympathy. But they also deserve to be informed of the truth.

Unfortunately, it seems a lot of doctors don't even *know* the truth. When Herb went for his annual exam with his new, fresh-out-of-med school PCP, he told her my story. She said as far as she knew, opioid withdrawal symptoms should be gone after two weeks.

Two weeks!

If this is as far as doctors know, if this is what they're being taught in med school, they desperately need to know further. If getting off of opioids were this easy, our country would not be engulfed in an epidemic of painkiller addiction. People would not be switching to heroin and fentanyl and dying of overdoses.

CHAPTER 11

When, after weeks of spring rain, we finally woke up to sunshine, I loaded a cart with tools and a lawn chair and dragged it out to the edge of the woods. Yeah, I felt like scraped-up, not-quite-dead roadkill, but as a fourth-generation Oregonian, I was trying to obey the paramount Oregon rule: *If it's not raining, go outside.* If I waited for good weather and vibrant energy to match up, I might never again get out there to what I thought of as the solace of the trees, the place I think of whenever any of my meditation CDs instruct me to mentally go where I feel safe and happy.

I love this little forest we've grown. I'm proud of it. Herb probably planted two Doug firs to each one I managed, and for a couple of years he and Mary had mowed between the rows, but after that, these trees had been mine. On hot summer evenings when the house was brimming with teen angst, I would go out to this far field and kneel at each tree to pull away the weeds. As the trees grew thickly together, I began lopping off the lower branches and the shorter of any double leads. For a few years we cut our own Christmas trees from the plantation; then they grew too tall for our living room. One autumn we drove the pickup truck out for a thinning project, Herb taking a chainsaw to the trees I'd flagged. My job was to cut off the branches, drag the six-inch diameter trunks toward the truck to be cut into firewood.

Today I would torch a burn pile, and make what progress I could in cleaning up the flood-floated masses of woody debris left from the river's rising in the winter of 2012. I wouldn't push myself, though. I took a book, in case I needed to rest, and my cell phone. Figured I'd phone Aunt Catherine. Useless in so many ways, I hadn't lost the ability to listen.

I wadded the newspaper, tee-peed the kindling. It had been so wet, it took me two or three matches, but soon enough I was throwing the branches on the crackling fire, loving as always the way the flames seemed to do so much of the work. Exercise in the fresh air was supposed to help get endorphin production going and, lucky me, I had this favorite project right out my own door.

An hour into it, wrestling a thicket of prunings that had floated and caught against a couple of trees, I looked toward the road clearing and saw smoke coming from the garden cart. Shoot. I dropped the branches and hustled back. A spark had ignited my canvas bag. Snatching it up, I dumped out my phone and book and reading glasses, holding at arm's length the burning bag which bore the ancient Hawaiian shield logo of Kona Village.

Just a month after our last visit to this beloved and laid-back resort on the Big Island, it had been destroyed by a tsunami. We hadn't been back to Hawaii since. We were hoping this little home away from home of ours would rebuild soon and reopen.

I tossed the half-burned bag on the fire and watched the flames flare up through the logo. It seemed like a movie scene. I hoped it wasn't an omen.

Well, okay. Maybe catching the wrong stuff on fire was a message for me: time for a break. I dropped into the lawn chair and dialed Aunt Catherine's number. Mailbox full. Herb said she sometimes had trouble with this. I phoned him for help, not knowing if he was still at the house or gone into town.

In answering, he said he was pulling over in front of the Bank of America downtown.

"And look who's coming down the sidewalk pushing his bike. It's Miles."

"Seriously?" With Miles's deep interest in China, we'd been bracing ourselves to lose this particular child of ours to a life in Asia. Now he lived right here in town where we could run into him on the street. How cool was that?

I heard Herb call out, "Hey, Miles!" as I tossed a stick on the fire. "Come say hi to your mom."

I heard some brief joshing, then, "Hey, Mom."

"Hey, honey. How fun. So how are you doing?"

"Actually, I'm doing good. *Really* good."

Hmm. A hint of something in his voice. Something beyond good.

"Yeah? " I said tentatively, squinting up at the trees. "So, are you getting your wife pregnant?"

Disclaimer: Yes! This sounds appalling! Who talks like that? But remember, *he* was the one who'd been so shockingly up-front about this little adventure of theirs.

"Arrrhhhhhh." Miles emitted a wail of happy dismay. "I wasn't supposed to say anything, but we're going to the doctor Monday."

"Wait, what? You really think you are?"

"Well, yeah, maybe. Except Ziwei's not convinced."

"Did you do a home test?"

"Yeah. Three actually."

"And they were positive?"

"Yeah, but see, we had this figured out on the computer and the timing just doesn't seem right."

I burst out laughing. "Oh, my God. Do you know how many of those tests came up negative for us when we were trying to get you guys? I really think if you've had three positives I'd be pretty surprised if you weren't."

"Well, we weren't going to tell anybody until we were absolutely sure."

"Oh, honey." I was weepy with delight now. "I'm sorry if this is going to upset Ziwei, but I'm glad I found out, because this is just the greatest thing ever. And I've been pretty desperate for good news. I can't stand thinking you'd have kept this from me for one minute."

"Okay, but don't say anything yet, okay?"

"Okay."

"Maybe it's hard for us to believe because Mom, it worked the *first time*. You had us so scared." (Apparently I hadn't been keeping my mouth shut on the subject as well as I'd been wanting to imagine.) "Hey, if I'd known I could control it like this, I never would have set my kid up for a Christmas birthday!"

I was laughing and crying at the same time as I got off the phone.

Seriously, I could not think of one other piece of news anyone could have delivered that would have been cause for greater joy.

I raked the fire together to burn down and loaded up the cart. Dragging it behind me, head down, I focused on the profusion of perky little daisies popping up through the grass along the path. Pure white with yellow centers against the fresh green grass. They were beautiful. I could register that. The sky was blue. Life was good. Wonderful things were coming our way.

And yet, physically, I still felt terrible.

This proves it, I thought.

I was not just some sad-sack person who only needed a bit of good news to spark her back to life. I was still very much in the grip of opioid withdrawal.

If anything, I felt a flutter of low-grade panic.

I was going to be a grandmother.

I had to get well.

Although we were still sworn to secrecy as far as the rest of the world, Miles had promised an announcement to Mary, Will, and Jaci at an inaugural Mother's Day gathering at the Kings Valley cabin.

We'd expected at least the tapping of a glass, a clearing of his throat. Instead, sotto voice, Miles just tossed it off:

"Ziwei won't be having a Mimosa because she's pregnant."

One stunned beat and everyone erupted into cheers.

Later during the brunch of Eggs Benedict (thank you, Mary and Jaci) and mellowed by his own Mimosa, this firstborn son of ours delivered a line rare and memorable for him for its complete lack of irony.

"Yep," he said, with nothing but the calmest conviction, "it's going to be the most awesome baby ever."

Honestly, I did *not* rub Herb's face in it, the fact that, see, they *were* going to need that bigger house.

I just got busy. I had already been emailing Clare with fair intensity on the subject of Willamette Landing. She knew the restrictions Herb had placed on me, that I was not to say anything to Miles and Ziwei in the absence of an announcement of a pregnancy. And now I was trying to operate under *their* restrictions, that their thrilling news not yet be made public.

My first email to Clare after hearing that a house with a bathtub would indeed be needed contained several direct questions about Willamette Landing houses and concluded with **Inquiring minds want to know!** And a wink icon. I'm guessing she got it.

I'd grown enamored of an impressive Willamette Landing home, the upper bedroom windows of which afforded a rare and expansive view of the river. It reminded me of how I'd written the ending of *Children of the River*, Sundara and Jonathan gazing at the Willamette together.....*stretching before them clear to the horizon, broad and inviting, shimmering with hope.*

To my everlasting delight, my son and his wife make excellent doubles for these characters I had invented around the time Miles was just two and Ziwei was splashing in the shallows of the Li River in Yangshuo, China. I wondered if it could be a sign this was the right house, the fact that I could so easily picture them holding up an early-waking baby to see the sunrise over the river, this real-life couple miraculously come together from opposite sides of the world.

To demonstrate to Herb that I was not entirely out of my romantic mind, however, I decided to drop in at the open house of one of Clare's own Willamette Landing listings, a more practically sized (and priced) house. Also, this would be supportive of Clare, I thought—help add to the sense of more people being interested in her listing, maybe stir up a competitive vibe.

As soon as I walked into the house by the park, though, all ulterior motives fell away. I took in the high ceilings, the south-facing bank of windows onto the backyard, the upgraded wood floors, and knew this sweet house could be just the one for Miles and Ziwei. What wasn't to love? The upstairs featured four rooms, one already decorated as a nursery, opening out onto a large central hallway, perfect for walking a crying baby at night. I saw my son like a lovely apparition of the future, bounce-walking the baby past me, patting him on the back.

I shut my eyes. Yes, this place would do nicely.

I walked out with a flyer.

I timed the drive back to our place. Five minutes. Couldn't beat it.

A few weeks later I emailed Clare the need for us to do lunch. **We have IMPORTANT things to discuss.** Another wink icon.

No! she wrote back. **Yes??**

Clare and I began quietly plotting the staging and sale of the Jackson Avenue bungalow. Pure craziness, adding the prepping of another house to our summer's work load, but Clare felt confident our little cream puff—real estate lingo, she told me, for such sweetly perfect cottages—would sell promptly. Not listing it until the end of the summer didn't scare her a bit.

She arranged a tour of available Willamette Landing houses with Miles and Ziwei, and I was thrilled when Miles invited us along to give advice. I felt horrid at the appointed hour, stiff and achy, but I was not about to miss this boots-on-the-ground house hunt. We looked, we took pictures, we went out to dinner afterwards. We discussed and debated. I would have said the whole thing went swimmingly, but what do I know? The next day we heard from Miles all the things Ziwei *hadn't* liked about various houses but, in her Chinese way, had been too reticent to mention in front of her elders.

Around and around the two of them went until they finally agreed upon the house to pursue. Ziwei surprised us all by rising to the occasion with the sort of steely, Chinese-style bargaining for which none of the rest of us had the stomach. Pearl in the palm, jewel of a daughter-in-law, I'm sure her stubborn skills honed in the markets of Yangshuo and Beijing ended up saving our son thousands.

They had circled back and would now be the new owners of the sweet little house by the park. The one just minutes from Wake Robin Farm.

CHAPTER 12

Eighty miles north, Will's Portland house now awaited our attention, and picturing our upcoming happy-family work parties had me cautiously excited. Herb would enjoy his most favorite sort of project, hauling plants from the nursery to re-do the yard. I'd have the satisfaction of painting over the cold taupe walls with a pale, glowing gold. And Will? Will could fetch lunch from the nearby eateries between bouts of cheerfully packing up his household goods in preparation for his amazing new life in Bend.

Nice, right? But nobody was giving me final script approval. Call re-write! Which idiot authorized the stupid changes we ended up trying to enact?

Maybe if Will had known how fast he'd land on his feet in Bend, maybe if he'd had more faith in his future, he'd have at least been able to mount some semblance of energy.

But he didn't. And maybe even more than his father, Will regards any kind of change with grave trepidation. He'd already had a rocky year. His three-year relationship had gone south. Or, more accurately, east to Colorado.

We arrived for the first of the half-dozen stints of rehab to find him pouting on the beer-stained sofa like a darkly roiling storm cloud.

I couldn't stand it. Many hands make light work, but the pair attached to Will wasn't looking promising. I was in no mood for coaxing.

Pick a room, any room, I remember thinking. *Just get started.* I went upstairs to the one bedroom cleared of furniture. At least the trashed carpet made an easy drop cloth. I pried open the paint, stirred, slopped some in the tray and started rolling "Michigan Dune" on the walls and ceiling.

A trip a couple weeks later involved me painting while overseeing the professional installation of the new kitchen counters. To paint the dining room, I had piled everything on the table and thrown a tarp over it. I hadn't reckoned on all the litter boxes though. Will's cats, of whom he was charmingly fond, seemed to need two in each room—nervous bladders or something—and horsing the ladders around them was a huge pain.

At one point I looked out the sliding French doors and saw Will standing in the corner of the backyard, a hose languidly draped over his hand. He looked so sad, so bored. I knew this was hard, and I felt for him. I wished I could make it better, kiss the boo-boo. But he was twenty-seven, in theory, an adult. We'd both had bad years. Unfortunately I was totally shorting out on whatever neurotransmitters it required to come off as a nurturing mom.

Stumbling in the litter box again, I thought, *I can't do this. I* **won't** *do this. And they can't make me.*

"This isn't going to work," I told Herb. "I'm not coming back to paint until Will moves out."

And I stuck to that.

I was not sleeping well. I'd wake in the middle of the night, and while I waited for my half-tab of Xanax to kick in, I'd surf the internet for help, for stories. The various opioid withdrawal sites began to pop up with helpful little reminders: *You last visited this site on 3/14. You last visited this site on 5/20.* And finally, a bit dismayingly, they gave up counting. *You have visited this site many times.*

One night in June I stumbled onto a site I hadn't seen before, one dealing with what is known as post-acute withdrawal syndrome. It delivered this shocking bolt:

Post-acute withdrawal usually lasts for two years.

Oh, my God. Tell me it's not true. You mean I'm only six months into this? I still have a year and a half to go?

At my age, two years seemed like a significant percentage of the time I probably had left on earth. I couldn't bear the thought of spending any more of it feeling like this, trying to live my life like I had a chronic case of the flu.

The article employed the metaphor of your brain working like a set of springs. Drug use depresses the production of certain neurotransmitters. When you stop the drugs, the springs pop up, producing symptoms. Then they bounce back and forth until they eventually regain equilibrium. Until then, these were your symptoms:

- Mood swings

- Anxiety

- Irritability

- Tiredness

- Variable energy

- Low enthusiasm

- Variable concentration

- Disturbed sleep

Bingo. Bingo. Bingo all the way down the list. Also, I had the weird pain in the back of my legs and the stabbing in my cheek.

The article explained the rollercoaster nature of post acute withdrawal which had so baffled me in the beginning. How come every time I thought I was well I'd just get sick again? Apparently that was the nature of the beast.

I forwarded this article to my mother and all three kids as a sort of plea for understanding.

The kids never commented and my mother wrote only this: **Wow, that's a really depressing article. I don't know what to say. I'm afraid whatever I say will be wrong so better left unsaid.**

Thank God I woke up with a little bit of energy on Will's moving day. With the house cleared, I could finally get started, and maybe this project could help get my endorphins pumping again. I wanted to see it sell so fast it would make Herb's head spin. I wanted validation for my foresight in the choice of this 1907 charmer.

I had my usual little notebook of To-Do lists, the whole house-painting project broken down into psychologically manage-able parts: **Choose colors....Buy paint....Paint upstairs bedroom first coat...Second coat...** Surely crossing off a few things would help quell my anxiety about meeting the deadline we had with the Realtor for listing the property.

Will's move was painstakingly planned. A small rental van had been reserved and would be waiting in Portland. Herb and I would drive to Portland, then he and Will would load the van, load Will's car, and the two of them would caravan around the flanks of Mount Hood and down 97 to Will's new rental duplex in Bend. Herb would stay there overnight and take the hopping flight from the Redmond airport back to PDX, where I would pick him up in the morning, having stayed the night by myself at the Best Western at the Meadows.

What could go wrong?

As we passed Salem on I-5, Will called.

"Mom, I just want to kind of warn you that I don't have every-thing *quite* packed up yet. So don't get all upset when you walk in."

"Don't worry," I assured him. "We'll work it out." I was practi-cally humming the old Mighty Mouse cartoon theme song, *HERE… we come….to save the daaay!* And Will had sounded upbeat. How bad could it be?

Unfortunately, bad. Very bad. Despite Will's well-intentioned warning, a wave of dismay flattened me when I walked into the house on North Syracuse Street. Any floor space not occupied by a box was strewn with items yet *un*-boxed. The kitchen overflowed with bottles, plastic, and everything else that should have long since been collected by Portland's extensive recycling program.

I'm sorry, I was disgusted. How many hours had I already spent on the phone with this kid, repeatedly talking him down from his pre-move jitters?

"Make a list," I'd told him when he'd called, at a loss as to how to pack up eight years of his life. "Break the whole thing down into small parts." I explained how I'd never dream of putting **Write Novel** on any To-Do list of mine. My list instead would say: **Write: Mon— Tues—Weds—Thurs—Fri,** and I'd cross off the days as I kept my promise to myself. "So yours could be like **Take a load to the dump. Get rid of the recycling.** And be sure to put some fun things on the list too, like **Sit in the hot tub.**"

"Yeah, I'm going to do that right now."

"No, honey, no! That's the *reward.* You let yourself do that *after* you've done some icky part."

After every one of these calls, I'd express my dire reservations to Herb.

"I'm telling you, honey, he's heading for a meltdown."

"He'll have it together," Herb kept saying. "Your trouble is you're getting him mixed up with Miles. Will isn't Miles."

Like I would ever confuse the two.

As a child, Miles argued the ridiculousness of the handshake as a social custom, while Will delighted in learning how to give grownups the glad hand. While Miles never saw the point of flattery, Will started practicing it at an almost frighteningly early age.

I remember once wrestling to diaper him on the change table. (Kids, this was the olden days, and we were conscientiously avoiding disposables, so please picture the effort it takes to not stab the little wriggler with pointy pins.) Noticing my harried frustration, baby Willie began using to great advantage what was probably his only word at the time.

"Mommeeee," he cajoled me with his winning smile, batting his big brown eyes. "Mommeee, Mommmeeee."

Wow. Kid's lucky I didn't step back in shock and let him roll off the table. I couldn't have been more startled by this precocious charm than if the cat had started singing "Won't You Be My Neighbor?" along with Mr. Rogers.

Also, Will had always been our organized son. The one who'd jump through whatever hoops were required. He did his high school homework at the crack of dawn and turned it in on time. He was the only one in the family who didn't breeze through books for pleasure, but his grades and SAT scores earned him a nice scholarship at UP. Once there, he doggedly stayed on the Dean's List in order to keep that money coming.

His sibs, in contrast, were forever hearing the beat of a different drummer. We would never forget how Miles stalled on packing for the cross country trip to his first (and, as it turned out, only) year at Hampshire College in Amherst, Massachusetts. Our reward for assiduously *not* helicoptering was a kid with a massive migraine on the day before leaving, nothing packed, much less shipped. I remember Herb gathering up the scattered contents of Miles's bedroom floor and just tossing it all willy-nilly into various cardboard shipping boxes.

That's what Herb meant when he said Will wasn't Miles.

But I'm the one who'd been fielding phone calls from this younger son, and I'd been vocal about my worries. Now, surveying all this dirt and disorganization, I wasn't one bit happy to have my skepticism confirmed.

"Is your bedroom at least cleared out?" I asked Will.

Those big brown eyes turned away from mine. "Yeah."

So this is what we'd come to—Darling Willie, fresh out of charm.

"Okay, I'm going upstairs to start painting." I looked at Herb. "I'm gonna let you guys deal with this."

In the upstairs bathroom I found a huge stack of old newspapers. Honestly, had Will paid any attention at all to my house-packing tutorials? I hugged the bundle to my chest, went out to the stairwell and dropped it in a straight shot over the railing to the hall by the front door. It landed with a satisfying smack, the papers fanning out.

Focus, *focus*. I put my iPod on angry Bonnie Raitt (men!) and started spackling the dozens of holes where tacks had held Will's soccer team scarves and ski posters to the walls. Then I began rolling on the pale paint I hoped would cover the dark green left by the former owner that made this room into such a cave. Obviously it would take several coats.

Shoot. I did not feel good. My legs ached. What energy I did have felt nervously manic, without strength or foundation. I remembered another piece of advice the acupuncture doctor Rose Tian had given me. "Try not to get too tired."

Right. And just how many hours of painting did I have ahead of me before this house would be ready for market?

I was only on the second wall past the ceiling when Herb carefully opened the door.

"Okay, here's the thing," he said. "Will's stuff isn't all going to fit into the truck, but—"

I lowered my roller, narrowed my eyes.

"But wait, wait…I have a plan. He can drive back next week for the rest. In the meantime, I'll just pile it neatly in the middle of the living room."

"Oh, no you won't. The whole point of waiting until he was out to start painting is because you can't expect somebody to have to work around that. If we were paying somebody else to do it, they wouldn't even set foot in the place until we had all that crap out of here. And I've been trying to warn you this was going to happen. Why should I have to pay the price?"

Herb popped his jaw. "Okay, so what's *your* great idea?"

"Simple. You cash in that plane ticket and he drives you back to Portland tomorrow and gets his second load."

"But I thought you'd rather not deal with him. Wouldn't you rather he came back when we're not here?"

"Herb! How's he supposed to learn anything? Isn't this one of those suffering-the-consequence-of-his-actions type things? If he'd packed up in time he'd have figured out you needed a bigger truck. We're his parents. It's not our job to find ways to let him off the hook all the time just because that's easier for us."

I could see Herb mentally casting around for another argument to bolster his case. Here's what he came up with: "But look how much later it'd be before I got back to help you with the work."

Scare me to death. To my mind, the work cut out for me in painting far exceeded what was slated for him on his landscape rehab.

"If I don't have to drive over and pick you up at the airport," I carefully countered, "I can come straight here from the motel in the morning and be at work that much faster." Diplomatic, right? At least considering what I was actually thinking.

Herb frowned. "But what about his cats? He's not going to want to leave them alone in a strange place."

I squeezed my eyes tight. The pain in my cheek stabbed. The cats? The cats who were on Prozac? Hey, I'd already had to pop a Xanax just to stay calm enough to get started here this morning. I was this kid's *mother*. Could I at least get equal consideration with Pepe and Sunny?

"You just think about that," Herb said, going out, his tone indicating I ought to feel guilty for even considering such cruelty to beloved pets.

In the end they bought my plan. Probably didn't dare not, the scary way I was acting.

The picture I took of Will in the empty living room gives evidence of me trying to make something positive of his exit. He grins gamely as he holds in each hand a cat in a carrier bought specifically for this journey.

But the rest of my memories of myself at the house on Syracuse Street all seem charged with my simmering rage. I see myself storming up the stairs that day he left, turning back to yell from the landing, shaking in fatigue and frustration, using words I'd never before directed at anyone, especially not my own child.

"Will, for God's sake, just get in the fucking truck and drive!"

I have no specific memory of their return the next day or what was said. I remember only lying flat on the back lawn, eyes shut, face to the sky, thinking, *I can't do this. Everything hurts. I'll never get all this work done and those two are no help at all. I wish I were anywhere but here, shackled to those two men, my husband and my son.*

If the ground had obligingly opened up, I'd have crawled right in and pulled the turf over my head.

But it was me who'd agitated to buy this house eight years ago and ultimately take on this project. I'd made this bed and now I had to lie in it.

Above ground.

I've never been a person at the mercy of food cravings. Even pregnant I didn't experience the weird dietary preferences detailed in female folklore. I noticed only my brain's command to eat. *Eat a lot!* Especially carrying the twins. Not being in any way a foodie, it actually bored me, how much time I had to devote to figuring out how to appease the Appetite Gods constantly demanding I chow down.

Same on prednisone. I'd been alerted weight gain could be a side effect of this steroid, but hey, no worries. I couldn't gain weight if I didn't up my caloric intake, right?

Ha! This powerful drug had no trouble completely and immediately overriding my best conscious intentions. I stuffed my face; in ten days, I gained five pounds.

I also remember back in college when, after my first major knee surgery, my appetite disappeared. I couldn't make myself eat. Skeletal at ninety-five pounds, I was under no anorexic delusion that ribs-clearly-delineated was an attractive look. I was then prescribed birth control pills to restart my periods—a bad idea, as it turned out, but at nineteen, I was still blindly doing whatever any certified M.D. told me to. On hormones, my brain suddenly insisted **Eat! Eat a lot! Get out of the dorm and get an apartment so you can make Bisquick coffee cake with brown sugar topping!** Since no normal thought of mine ever involved a cooking project, I knew something weird was going on.

When I showed up at Thanksgiving, having put on twenty pounds in five months, my brother was astonished. "You're fat!"

It haunts me still, the fact that when he blurted this out I weighed 115 pounds. Short of a terminal wasting illness, I'm pretty sure I'll never see 115 again.

So while I've always had a sense of brain chemicals affecting appetite, I'd never had a craving for anything specific.

Until now.

Great Harvest Bakery on the Corvallis riverfront makes a popular loaf of bread called Apple Crunch. Get real, though—it's cake; deep denial required to kid yourself otherwise. Big, spongy, and thickly crusted with brown sugar. Comes unsliced. You're free to hack off a huge chunk. Go ahead, slather it with butter. Why not? We're so far beyond worrying about the calorie count here. Let that concern remain in some other healthy universe where brains presumably aren't on fire, screaming to be calmed.

It was all about the serotonin. Carbs, apparently, help release it in your brain. With my sickly neurotransmitters, I found I absolutely *craved* this fix. I would be driving home from errands and suddenly jerk the wheel for a detour down to the riverfront. Or at home, suffering on the sofa, I would remember the bread and rise like a zombie, get my car keys and steer straight for Great Harvest Bakery. I always felt like a true addict walking in.

The fresh-faced young people working there unfailingly articulated the shop's generous policy. "Do you want to try a sample slice today?"

I always shook my head *no*, smiling sheepishly, knowing that the minute I got home I would be stuffing down a full quarter of the sugary loaf.

As if by casually waving off the chance of a faster fix I was somehow retaining a small crumb of control, some last little vestige of dignity.

Our VISA bills show seven trips to Portland in those June weeks of 2013, each with two or three nights at the Best Western. Each work day was the same; I never had any energy to start with and from there proceeded to utter exhaustion. Three o'clock invariably found me in crisis, crouched on a stool in front of the altar of Will's left-behind microwave, hot, sweaty and weeping, waiting for the Xanax to kick in, waiting to butter up the heated Apple Crunch bread and cram it down.

I wasn't proud to be using the crutch of Xanax, but this wasn't like some case of vague, free-floating anxiety. I had a concrete explanation for falling apart. And I never sneaked it. I always reported it to Herb, and dutifully recorded it on the chart I kept.

"I think it's an entirely appropriate use of it," he'd always say.

No mystery, his attitude. As the guy who had to deal with me, I couldn't blame him for appreciating how this drug could stop a total freakout in its tracks. And I was a woman with work to do. We had a deadline.

"I don't understand why this isn't any fun," I said more than once. "I've been looking forward to this for so long."

"Well, it's not a fun thing," Herb tried to convince me.

But I vaguely knew this wasn't right. Housing rehab was never fun for him, true, but secretly he was enjoying the gardening, and didn't my old self used to get more satisfaction out of watching a creative transformation such as this take shape under my own hands? But then, I was hardly the person to trust in remembering who I used to be or how I'd felt about anything. I had *lost* that girl.

Now, looking back, I understand that six months off of opioids, I had arrived at perhaps the peak period for intensified anhedonia, the inability to experience pleasure. So of course there was nothing good in this project for me. There was nothing good in *anything* for me. My life felt like that of an 18th century indentured servant, shackled to endless hours of grueling work without respite.

And even without half our team being in drug withdrawal, wouldn't any two people trying to work together under the pressure of preparing properties for sale be going at least a little bit crazy? It's not like we were just sitting back and getting ready to cash in, after all. This was a concerted effort to retire all these mortgages and simplify our life. It wasn't going to pencil out if we didn't do the prep work necessary to earn decent sale prices.

A rare June heat wave wasn't helping. This is Oregon, remember. Air conditioning is not omnipresent. We couldn't just flip a switch.

"We're doing okay," Herb kept saying, always pressing his hands on my shoulders as if I were in danger of flying off when, actually, doing this made my knees want to buckle. "Aren't we on schedule for what we told the Realtor about the date to go on the market?"

"I guess," I'd lie, trying to be civil. I'd been huffing and puffing up and down the stairs, up and down the ladders, pushing it every minute, racing the clock. What I really felt, but didn't say, was that if I were tackling the work cut out for me at his steady but laid-back pace, no, we would *not* finish.

Occasionally my afternoon meltdowns took a different twist. After the new carpet was installed upstairs, I'd sometimes lie flat on my back in one of the bedrooms with my iPod and try to zone out to one of my hypnosis tracks. Mixed results, at best. I'd often awaken with my whole body in a giant cramp, or in the mental grip of a horrific nightmare.

Once, in one of those bedrooms, hysterical with fatigue, I remember Herb trying to hold me, calm me while I just kept sobbing that I was broken, so broken, my brain was broken.

"No, it's not. You're not broken. You're getting better all the time."

He *wished*. Jesus, the man was completely deluded.

For dinner we'd clean up enough to go over to Fishwife Seafood on Lombard. We're both such creatures of habit, drawn to comfortable familiarity. Every evening I'd gratefully drop into the same red vinyl seat by the window and order one crab dish or another plus a Margarita.

Herb drank iced tea. He'd given up alcohol back about the time Laura Bush kicked George's butt on the subject. No Twelve Step. No groups. He's no more of a joiner than I am. He just quit and never looked back, a couple of times in later years expressing gratitude for my calling him on this. Generously, he never begrudged me my one drink a day, a habit I'd taken up long after he quit, when I read somewhere that this actually conferred health benefits, and that if you were the rare person who could stick to just one, you were golden.

Well, I could do that. And I loved my Margaritas those nights in Portland. They revived me out of my sense of hopelessness. Fought back the fatigue so that I could go back to the house after dinner and at least do a little straightening up.

Then, completely out of steam, we'd head for the Best Western, where I would sink my paralyzed body in a hot bath. We checked on our chicks by email—Will's job hunt and Miles's adventures in mortgage seeking—joking that Mary seemed to be helping out by somehow managing to conduct her life these days without any advice from us whatsoever.

Then we'd crash.

Next day, get up and do it again.

In Bend, storm cloud Will morphed back into our sunny boy, once more a family bright spot. A week after moving, he'd answered an open call to work the bottling line at one of the ubiquitous handcraft breweries of Central Oregon. With seventy-five people in line ahead of him and twenty-five behind, odds for landing one of the two spots available seemed slim. He said he thought of bagging it, but then decided, *what the hell,* and stuck it out.

He got the job.

"So let's get this straight," the twin brothers interviewing him reportedly said. "You don't know anybody in Bend and you didn't have a job already lined up? You just moved to Bend to ski?"

"That's about the size of it."

Made perfect sense to them. Welcome aboard, bro!

Finally, we almost had the Portland house ready. Every whiff of *college kid* had been eradicated and the place looked beautiful. The French sliders opened to a backyard brought amazingly to life by green-thumbed Herb. The timing on the blooming of the roses, lilies and geraniums was going to be perfect.

Our staging would be minimal, Herb having declared from the outset he wasn't hauling truckloads of furniture from Corvallis. Fine by me. I'd hung carefully selected prints and paintings on certain walls and left Will's dining table under the low hanging light fixture. Over it I draped, for luck and because it looked perfect, the tablecloth I'd bought from a street vendor at the Great Wall of China.

In the living room we rolled out the antique carpet we'd scored for a song at an auction, and in a smaller adjacent room I'd placed a new carpet I'd bought on sale specifically for this staging. I'm sure the brain chemicals of pleasure hummed when I laid it over the imperfect spot on the wood floors and saw how it picked up the colors of the floral print I'd hung in that room. Just one tiny brain reward hit of *Damn, I'm good!*

In case our lives weren't complicated enough with putting this house on the market and getting the Jackson Avenue bungalow ready for the same, we were also trying to un-burden ourselves of a house we'd owned for over ten years at a Cascade mountain resort called Black Butte Ranch. We had hustled through the final prep and cleaning on that place right before my surgery, and it had been on the hibernating winter market since Labor Day.

Now our Black Butte Realtor alerted us he was expecting an offer on the place, which set off a whole new round of speculation regarding the upcoming priorities on our master To-Do list.

The night before our last day of work in Portland, lying in bed at the Best Western, we had trouble sleeping, Herb saying he couldn't stop trying to figure out the best way to pack up the paintings at Black Butte to get them home safely. When we both woke at the crack of dawn, we decided to get up and get going. Horses smelling the barn.

It was just six a.m. when we reached the house on Syracuse Street.

"Hey, the gate's open," I said when we got out of the truck.

"Yeah," Herb said darkly. "That's not all."

He'd seen it before me—the smashed-in door.

"Oh, no," I said, "Oh, no."

A break-in.

Herb pushed into the small office off the front porch where we'd gathered all the tools and paints, planning to move them out today.

"Great," he muttered. "How am I supposed to finish up? They took my whole toolbox."

"My rug!" The little piece de resistance was gone.

Herb moved ahead of me to the living room. "Got the other one, too," he called back. "Oh wait, no. Rolled it up but maybe it was too heavy."

I exhaled. "Well, that's good anyway."

"Got the M3P player."

I sank to sitting on the floor, I was shaking so badly. Lucky enough to have never before been the victim of a break-in, I now understood in an instant what people meant saying they felt violated. And this wasn't even my personal space. I'd never even slept here. And I suddenly knew, too, how literally people used that other word: *shaken*.

So, what else had been stolen? I rose, and we wandered the house, taking inventory, calling to each other the tentative good news of each item still remaining. In the upstairs hall I'd hung a gorgeous painting of lush pink peonies done by Ziwei's mother in China. Still there. Relief.

In the end, an almost-full bottle of tequila was the only additional item missing. Funny. It's not like we stock a home bar. The only reason that bottle was sitting on an open kitchen shelf was because I'd given myself the treat of a single Margarita on the Fourth of the July, a day when we'd been working while others partied and Fishwife Seafood was closed.

Alcohol being nabbed is what put the idea of addiction in my head. Will had mentioned certain areas near this North Portland neighborhood where addicts were known to congregate, and we'd seen sketchy types swooping through on bikes. Guy probably grabbed whatever could be most quickly turned into money to feed whatever habit he had going. Maybe he was even hooked on the very stuff I was trying to recover from: Oxycodone.

Poor jerk.

I looked around. Gallons of leftover paint with the pry key right there at hand. How easy it would have been to splash paint in an angry arc all over everything, ruining my work. At least this wasn't vandalism.

Thanks, I thought. *Thanks for what you didn't do.*

Still, it was crushing. The Realtor would be coming in a couple of hours. Weirdly, I felt...*ashamed.* We were offering this house up as a beautiful place for a family to live. Now it seemed the house itself had been violated. Was that something you were supposed to tell people as a disclaimer?

I took a Xanax.

Herb was so good, so steady.

"We're not going to let this idiot stop us from putting the house on the market, right? Better get in and wrap it up."

He left me sitting on the floor with a wad of steel wool and a can of wood restorer and drove off to buy new tools. When he came back, he brought a cheap new M3P player for the music he knew I needed, his playlist of sentimental country songs featuring happy endings and lines that rhymed wife with life. I was certainly not a person safely left alone with my own dark train of thought.

Then he set to rebuilding the doorframe.

When the Realtor showed, he didn't seem particularly distressed with the news of the break-in. It was still a beautiful house; he wasn't anticipating any trouble selling it.

I seemed to be taking this much harder than either of these two men.

For them it was apparently a small speed bump. For me it was a grimly memorable, three-Xanax catastrophe of a final day's work.

CHAPTER 13

———————————

I'd been to baby showers; I knew the drill. As the grandmother of this baby-to-be, I was expected to show up with something lovingly handmade. My obligation, my privilege. I'd been looking forward to it for years.

This should be the most special quilt I'd ever made. I went on Etsy and ran a search for fabrics with Asian motifs, an on-line activity as much fun for me as house hunting. I settled on a pattern of pig-tailed Chinese children twirling parasols, flying kites and spinning tops against a panorama dotted with arched bridges and pagodas, all done in what seemed to be a popular Chinese color combination of red, pink, turquoise, lime green and black.

Brilliant idea: I'd cut the pieces to frame each little scene.

Except—a dark thought slithered in—*Miles will probably give me a hard time about it.* I'm forever in trouble with him for my long-time romance with aspects of Chinese culture he considers false. Or *something.*

When the Etsy package arrived, I opened it with a certain trepidation. I could hear him mocking me, see the look on his face. *Mom,
this is NOT how it is for kids in China!*

So? I thought, concocting my defenses in advance to this crit-
icism that so far existed only in the bleakness of my sick mind. *Kids
here don't dress like Little Bo Peep, and we still do nursery drawings of
girls in poofy skirts.*

And further, grimmer still—*So what do you want? A fabric
printed with bloody depictions of the Cultural Revolution?*

Too bad everything always had to be so difficult with him. I
just wanted to do a little grandma project that would make me feel
better. But Miles being Miles, I was too scared.

I tossed the packet of fabric in the messy, catchall sewing room
and shut the door.

Flailing around, desperate for some kind of reassurance,
I phoned Dr. Herrick. Yes, as Herb had pointed out, he was now
retired. But he had such a reputation for kindness—I couldn't resist
a chance of hearing something of comfort. And, after all, we went to
the same church. Wasn't that supposed to count for something?

"I just need some stories," I pleaded to him. "I want to hear about
somebody like me who went through this and eventually got well."

"But you're the storyteller."

A reference to me being a writer, I guess.

"I don't know *this* story, though. I need somebody like you
to tell me what happens when somebody like me gets accidentally
addicted."

"You're not addicted," he said with what sounded like a hint of
impatience. "You're physically dependent."

"I know, I know." We'd been through this after he'd prescribed me Xanax for our trip to China and I'd had such a hard time getting off of it afterward. "But what difference does it make?"

"Oh, Linda, if you were an addict, you'd be stealing pills out of other people's medicine cabinets. You'd be doing anything to get your hands on more."

Great. I stared out my office window at the oak tree branches. He was giving me permission to not label myself a drug addict. Presumably I was supposed to feel validated by the fact that he was assuming I hadn't engaged in the morally reprehensible acts generally associated with addiction.

I just couldn't see how that was actually supposed to help.

"I'm having all the same withdrawal symptoms as any addict," I pointed out. I don't think my body cares what we're calling it. And I just feel so…..alone. Have you had other patients like me who went through this?"

"You're not alone," he said. "I can think of a couple of people who had to take opioids after surgery and had a hard time getting off."

"Well, what happened? How long did it take?"

"Oh….they had to struggle for quite awhile."

Doctors are so schooled in *not* being storytellers. Everything must be kept in confidence. Privacy must be guarded. Never mind if a story would help the next poor soul.

So he says I'm not alone. But only if you call it "not alone" when a prisoner learns there may be others similarly locked in solitary confinement in distant cells on the far side of the prison.

And "quite awhile." What did that mean? His deliberate vagueness made me feel he thought the honest answer—what, years?—might be too frightening to actually put into spoken words.

"We do have *some* good news," I finally offered. Dr. Herrick had actually had more office visits with Herb than with me, so I knew he'd be glad to hear this. "Herb's going to be a grandfather. You know he's going to love that."

"Oh, that's wonderful!" Seizing this happier topic with obvious relief, he expounded on the delights of grandparenthood.

When we hung up, I felt guiltily disconsolate. What I'd needed wasn't convincing on the idea of a grandchild being a good thing.

I was sorry I'd made the call. I'd be even sorrier later, remembering it.

On top of being pregnant, Ziwei was suffering terrible grass seed allergies. She'd never had trouble in Beijing, with its notoriously dirty air, and yet when we'd brought her to live under the blue summer skies of Oregon, she'd landed in the grass seed capital of the world, and she was miserable.

I felt guilty. She needed all the family support we could muster.

We set a date for their move from the Jackson Avenue bungalow to their new Willamette Landing house: the first Saturday after they'd be handed the keys. Doing it on a weekend meant Mary could help. Lucky, we explained to Ziwei. She had married into a family in possession of a pick-up truck. This is how we do it in America when we're only moving across town. It's easy! It's exciting! A spiffy new house! Everybody will pitch in!

Ziwei balked. Already exhausted and overwhelmed, she didn't see how she and Miles could be packed up by that date. And anyway, to be fair, hadn't they paid rent through the following Wednesday?

To be fair? Oh, ouch. Pain in the brain, pain in the face. Team Mother-in-Law could not win in this clash of cultures. By American standards, my parenting model had already been slyly questioned by admirers of both the Jackson Avenue bungalow as well as the cottage I'd fixed up for Mary in Eugene.

"Well, I certainly hope they *appreciate* this."

"I never would have set my kids up like this."

"I hope you're charging them rent."

Nobody ever came right out with the S word, but you could hear it in their voices.

The American take on it seemed to be that I was *enabling* my kids by giving them a nicer house than they deserved for less rent than they ought to be paying.

But coming from China, Ziwei had never quite understood having to pay rent to her in-laws in the first place. In her culture, Miles let me know, a family well-fixed enough might simply buy a house outright for a young couple. Put it in the woman's name to boot.

Herb agreed the kids were difficult and annoying, but reminded me that in this conflict, we still had to be the grownups.

Got that. I'd been hearing this wise refrain of his for years. But our kids weren't teenagers anymore. Miles would be thirty-four in a month. Mary and Will were twenty-seven. Was there ever going to be a point where I could hope for reciprocal comfort and support from them?

I couldn't help remembering when Herb and I were at their stage of life. We'd only been married three years when my parents had a car accident that nearly killed my mother, ultimately keeping her in the hospital for the better part of a year. I was twenty-seven, Herb twenty-eight, teaching eighth-grade English. Every day after school we got in our little red truck and drove the hour to visit her at Salem Memorial Hospital. When she was transferred to the Oregon Health Sciences University in Portland, we cut our trips to three times a week, but still, her care and support dominated our lives. When I read the journal I kept during this time, I shudder at the way I'd thrown my fledgling marriage on my mother's sacrificial altar. Not that she demanded it; we gave it as her due. And Herb was a young hero even then. If this is what I needed to do for my mother, he was there for me.

But now, when I'd wandered across this barren plain, where were the ones I needed to see my distress and, as Linda Ronstadt used to sing, keep me from blowing away? Maybe it would have been different if I'd been in the hospital, hooked to IV lines. Instead I was walking around, looking well enough, I suppose. But my mental distress was....I want to use the word unbearable, but obviously I *did* bear it. I'm alive, writing this.

What a horror, though, that sick little never-shutting-up voice in my brain. *Are you noticing this?* it nagged at me. *Your children apparently do not love you the way you loved your mother.*

As the day set for moving approached, I saw it wasn't going to be the happy little family work party I'd started out envisioning when their offer on the Willamette Landing house was accepted. The memory of Will's moving day buzzed a warning and, in an act of self defense, I opted out. The fact that I was still sick in this weird, un-seeable way clearly didn't seem to be registering with anybody, and I was loathe to set myself up for a meltdown nobody would understand, much less forgive. I told Herb I would bring Thai take-out over to the new house at dinner. Me *not* there was better. People could focus on taking care of Ziwei. The pregnant card played so much better than the drug addict card.

Except, excuse me. Of course I'm not really a drug addict. Everyone can feel so much better knowing that. Nobody has to take time out of their lives to research rehab facilities. The kids aren't phoning each other, frantically trying to track me down after I've gone missing from wherever they've checked me in. I'm not showing up at the ER, making false claims of being assaulted and thus in need of pain meds. Nobody's physically restraining me, counting their own pills. Nobody's finding me overdosed and blue. Nobody's having to shoot me up with Narcan to jerk me back from the brink for one more try at staying clean. Nobody has to call 911.

So happy to be able to spare everybody this embarrassing label—drug addict.

But my body didn't care what we called it: I still felt like shit.

And sometimes I couldn't help the wistful thought that maybe if I *had* qualified as a true addict, I'd have rated some helpful attention. Even an intervention didn't sound too bad. At least everybody would have had to show up for me, gather together in a visible demonstration of love and concern.

But no, I didn't seem to be officially, dramatically, an addict. I was just a person with a baffling, who-could-possibly-say-the-right-thing-to-her type problem, ghostwalking among these people who were supposedly my family.

CHAPTER 14

The first time I ran away to the beach house on my own I stuck a post-a-note on the microwave: **Enjoy your vacation from me.**

I meant it. I was not Cute Enough to Keep. I was the Bitch of the World.

Driving north, I shocked myself by noticing how much better I felt every mile I put between my husband and myself. Wasn't I the one who always claimed there was nothing I'd rather do than climb in the truck with this guy and head off for a day's work in the forest?

Now I wanted to be alone; *had* to be.

My whole family was driving me crazy; Herb worst of all.

I fell in love with this guy the first time I laid eyes on his beautiful face across the dining table at Lewis & Clark College. Almost forty-five years later, I *still* love that face, and looking back over my life, I realize that other than the faces of my own newborn babies, there is no other person walking the earth whose face I can claim to recall from the very first moment I saw it.

But he has this habit that was ruining it for me. He continually pops his jaw, some kind of self-soothing mechanism, an inherited trait apparently, seeing how his beloved grandfather was also known for this quirk.

Now, every time I'd turn to look at him, just hoping for my usual hit of pleasure, he'd be popping his damned jaw like an old guy. He was stealing something from me! I wanted my handsome husband back!

"But it's entirely unconscious," he'd point out, as if that should give him a pass on this odious little tic that was making me want to scream.

If it weren't for remembering how terribly painful our fights were, these scenes would be funny, watching them like an old movie. So stupidly obvious. Irritability was number three on that list of symptoms of post-acute withdrawal I'd seen on-line, right after mood swings and anxiety. I was a walking, talking, flipping-out, textbook illustration of irritability.

And I knew this. The trouble was, I knew it with a compromised brain. I kept trying to think it through. Was Herb popping his jaw more than usual because I was stressing him out? Was my reaction exaggerated by the snarly state of my brain? After all, he'd been doing this forever and it hadn't ever flipped me out like this before.

Never veering an inch off the road of straight and steady, Herb could only find me completely baffling.

"Well, if you can't stand me," he'd say, "maybe you *should* leave."

Dimly, that didn't seem right. But my brain was so fogged. Before all this I'd have sworn we had a marriage for the ages. Rock solid. We'd been through so much together. Things anybody would call way more challenging than an annoyance with jaw popping.

Was this actually going to do us in? Could he really mean it, that I should leave?

I remember crying, saying I just didn't know where our marriage was headed. I was trying to picture the future and I couldn't see anything good. All we did together was work. Were we ever going to do anything fun?

"These houses were *your* projects," Herb would point out again. "Don't blame me we have to do all this work."

"I know, I know. But after. When we get done."

"What is it you want to do so bad?"

I thought. Nothing sounded fun to me, now or ever. I dredged up something that had appealed to me in the past.

"How about that class at Linn-Benton I told you about—Cowboy Dancing?"

He made a sour face. "Forget it."

"Come on. Why not? You like country music. It'd be fun."

He sighed. "Haven't we been through this?"

Oh, yes, we certainly had. Herb had always staunchly, proudly maintained his stance against dancing. He treasured his story of his mother signing him up at twelve for cotillion in Pacific Palisades, California, how he'd escape out the back door with his buddy to play away dance class time in the ravine.

"Don't forget," I said, "it's *your* music that made me think of this." Ian Tyson's cowboy songs had been one of the sound tracks of our lives. *Darlin', we haven't gone dancing, in such a long time now.....*

"Why can't you just do your belly dancing?"

Oh, yeah, he was all for that, especially when I came home in my swishy skirts, all flushed and whipped up.

"Maybe I want to dance with a *man*," I said. "Cowboy Dancing is a couples class. I don't think you'd be too happy if I started checking around who else might want to sign up with me."

He sat there—stubborn, silent.

Here's what I'd figured out about my husband quite awhile back: Herb did what Herb wanted to do. In so many ways what he wanted to do ended up making life better for a lot of people. We all benefitted from his green thumb, the home-grown fruits and vegetables he cooked into amazing meals, the apples pressed into cider. If somebody needed a shrub stuck in their yard, he was there. Were you snowed in? He'd bring firewood in his four-wheel drive. He was kind and generous, and if you were on his list and his skill set covered something you needed doing, well then, good for you.

But Herb Crew was determined not to dance. If you were his wife and you wanted to go Cowboy Dancing, you were—sorry, no better way to put it—shit-out-of-luck.

I felt surprisingly free, driving up good old scenic Highway 99W. In Monmouth I decided to pull over at Burgerville and get a Mocha Perk. I could do that! I was in the driver's seat. I didn't mind Herb always doing the driving, but I was pretty sure it never occurred to him how much control that gave him. He could take an unexplained detour for some errand and make me have to ask if I wanted a clue what was up. He could cruise past an intriguing-looking antiques shop and, a mile down the road, innocently ask, "Oh, did you want to stop there?"

So I was enjoying what passed, for me anyway, as a moment of defiant empowerment, standing in the Burgerville parking lot with my caffeinated milkshake.

A pack of bicyclists was arriving one by one for a pit stop, and I began chatting up the leader, who told me they were a club, out for a spin around the valley. He seemed a fit late-sixties.

"That really looks like fun," I said, pretty sure he'd never have guessed I was a wife who'd half an hour ago lit out on her husband, mad as hell. "I just got a new knee, so maybe I'll be able to do that one of these days."

I had a life, right? I had a future.

"Well check this," he said, rolling his bike closer, pulling up the stretchy hems of both legs of his lycra shorts to reveal the full length of the scars running up the center of each knee. "Got 'em both done in October."

"Wow." So, a month after me. It was July now. Ten months since my surgery. Only nine since his.

"I figured, why not have just one recovery. Get it over with."

"That's amazing."

"He is," said a woman who pulled up on her bike beside him. His wife? No, a fellow club member. Actually, it soon became apparent, more like his publicity agent.

"The Salem paper did a huge article about him," she said. "He's like the hospital's poster boy for rehab."

"Amazing," I said, a word I kept repeating as she continued with her accolades. This guy's story was what I'd had in mind for myself, to come out of this better than ever. A new, healthier me. Where had I gone wrong?

"Actually," I said, "I'm doing okay with my knee. What's been hard for me has been getting off the narcotics. I mean, I quit ages ago, but I'm still having all these withdrawal issues."

"Oh." He shrugged. "Well, I'm still on Vicodin." He bent and frowned at something in his bike spokes.

Uh-oh. So, just how much of this was going on? People taking narcotics after surgery and then never managing to stop? I wondered if the newspaper puff piece mentioned this. Probably not. Cycling was inspirational; Vicodin addiction, not so much.

"Whatever works, I guess." I'd offered my confession in hopes he'd have something helpful or encouraging to say about dealing with the effects of withdrawal. But he didn't have that story to tell. Not yet. And he was enjoying his bike ride. Being the hospital's star patient.

He wouldn't want to hear my take on it.

Maybe I was wising up: I kept my mouth shut.

The beach house had been my idea, my post-partum fantasy come true. Sitting there nursing two babies at the same time, staring out the window, I thought that if this is what I was going to be doing all the time, wouldn't it be nice to occasionally look out the window at a different scene? Crashing white ocean waves were always nice.

My grandfather had bought a cabin in Yachats during the Depression, and my affection for the place they named Ocean Crest had been the genesis of my book, *Someday I'll Laugh About This.* Herb and I had spent our honeymoon there, and tried to get toddler Miles over there whenever we could, most memorably finding our designated weekend coinciding with the Friday the Thirteenth Windstorm of 1981, when winds over a hundred-miles-an-hour violently vibrated the little cabin all night long. Power was out along the coast for days, and Herb was not amused at the way two-year-old Miles would not stay out of all the cooking pans strategically placed to catch the drips through the roof. I thought it was funny, but then, I wasn't the one on the roof trying to replace the blown-away shingles.

By the eighties, too many cousins were all trying to book time at Ocean Crest. I foresaw conflicts of ownership and maintenance looming. Maybe Herb and I ought to start our own tradition. Wouldn't he be happier patching shingles on his own beach house?

"Are you kidding?" he said. "Now? With two babies to deal with? This would be the very worst time in the world to be trying to do something like that."

I couldn't argue. But I couldn't stop scanning real estate ads in the *Oregonian* either. He kept explaining why this was such a horrible idea. I kept agreeing; I kept searching.

Finally he relented and humored me with a quick scouting trip to the coast. I was thrilled to be out of the house and actually going somewhere on this beautiful spring day. Even if it involved the juggling of nursing babies. Even if we had to be home before Miles got out of school at three.

When we passed the green Neskowin sign, I felt a buzz. I loved that name. My grandfather's story about the Yachats cabin had always been that he'd first looked for property in Neskowin, because that's where all the "toney" people went. (Loved it!) Only when the owner of Ocean Crest made him a Depression-era offer of desperation he couldn't refuse—$500—did he relinquish his dream of the little coastal town farther north.

The Neskowin Realtor I'd made an appointment with stood us up, so we drove directly into the little village—one adorable cottage after another, twisty shore pines arching so charmingly over the narrow lanes. Carrying Mary and Willie, we walked out onto the beach and looked south across the creek that fanned out around Proposal Rock. New homes lined the ocean front, but at a distance we could see three older-looking cottages in a row.

"That's what I had in mind," I said. "Those over there."

We loaded the babies back into their car seats and drove out to cross the creek at the highway bridge. Inconveniently, none of the three vintage houses were for sale (!) So naïve, this business of imagining we could just drop in and see which beloved family beach house we'd choose. Later I'd understand: these places weren't going on the market. These shingled roofs sheltered decades of memories that couldn't be bought. We'd have to find a place and start making our own.

At the end of the road, we got out and walked down the beach access path.

"Okay, *this* is where I'd want to be," Herb said, scanning the scene. "You could walk down to the creek, but mostly you'd be over here where it's quieter and away from the crowds at the park."

I murmured assent, careful to curb my enthusiasm. But, yay! He was sounding very much like a guy who might actually commit to buying a Neskowin beach house.

A few days later we had a call from a fellow in Neskowin who'd got wind of our search and thought we might be interested in the brand new beach-front house he'd been building. He was living in it, but only until he finished and sold it. We made a date to look, driving up on our way home from a weekend at Ocean Crest.

All three kids were past worn out by the time we made it to Neskowin and pulled up at this modest little house, so unprepossessing, we'd completely overlooked it on our earlier trip, even though it sat right on the stretch of beach Herb liked.

I hated the place. Not for its small size, but because of the builder's interpretation of having "lived lightly" in it. True, he'd hammered no picture-hanging holes in the walls. No, he'd just saturated every fiber of the horrid wall-to-wall carpeting and drapes with cigarette smoke that gave me an instant headache.

Professionally decorated, he proudly informed us. Later we'd learn the pro was his ex-wife. I looked around, trying to mask my dismay. The Formica countertops were a shade of orange that went out in the sixties and in 1986 had not yet come back around—except for this place. Each of the three small bedrooms had windows layered in chiffon and satin.

Who does that at a beach house? I'd hoped for a funky old place like Ocean Crest—the musty smell of curtains saturated with salty ocean air, not disgusting tobacco smoke.

But Herb was just standing in the living room, transfixed by the broad view of the ocean—the first outcroppings of Cascade Head to the left and, to the right, Proposal Rock and beyond, all the way to Cape Kiwanda at Pacific City.

Strapping the babies back in their car seats, I was exhausted and completely disappointed with the house, sorry I'd dragged everybody on this wild goose chase.

But Herb wasn't bummed at all. He liked it. "Location, location, location," he said as we pulled out onto Highway 101. The smoky curtains were an easy fix, he pointed out, and by the time we reached the crest of Cascade Head and were starting down the other side, it was Herb who'd convinced me this thirteen-hundred square foot house was the place for us.

I'll give him credit for that if he'll give me points for sensing this was not the worst time in the world to start this new tradition.

Actually, it turned out to be the best.

In the twenty-seven years we'd owned the beach house, I had never once fled there on my own.

Not until now.

And I was enjoying being there by myself. Nobody to set me off. No Xanax necessary.

Not that I felt physically well. I still had the horrid pain in my left sinus. My teeth felt weirdly tight. Trying to keep in mind that just because I had one thing—drug withdrawal—didn't mean I couldn't fall prey to some other ailment, I had Googled "tight teeth." A dentist, I learned, would probably be glad to shave off the edges to relieve this pressure. Well, no thanks. That sounded like the very sort of procedure somebody would be deeming painful enough to be urging narcotics on me. I remember hoping this was just my last weird withdrawal symptom which would soon go away on its own.

My friend Karen came to hang with me and hash out life and marriage and husbands. I told her about the bicyclist on Vicodin, because even before my surgery I'd been concerned about her long-term use of this opioid. I'd always let myself be reassured by her insistence that her pharmaceutical protocol was entirely by prescription. Now I thought, yeah? So what? So was mine. A doctor's Rx pad was clearly no protection against addiction; that prescription pad was more like a passport to hell. Karen was my friend. She's been on this stuff for six years. Didn't I owe her a warning?

"I read an article," I told her, "that said they're starting to realize narcotic painkillers aren't a good long term-prescription for fibromyalgia."

"Oh." She hesitated. "Well. I don't even know that I really have that. I just say fibromyalgia because it's something people recognize."

She started insisting I was only in withdrawal trouble because I'd disregarded my doctor's orders by taking just three weeks to taper. Then she pivoted, accusing me of lacking faith in her ability to go off the drugs. That really hurt her feelings (!)

"The proof's in the pudding," she said, with a vehemence that made no sense because... yeah, exactly. She'd already told me her doctors said she needed to start tapering off.

"But that's the thing," I said. "You're not going off."

"But I'm going to!" And then, as if anybody expecting her to detox indicated a gross misunderstanding of her busy life, she added, "Honestly, I have way too much going on this summer to even think about it."

Okay, this argument was going nowhere. I had promised I would make my case and then shut up. Never bring it up again. It wasn't until months later that I finally I saw: I couldn't keep this promise. We couldn't be friends now, couldn't simultaneously share the same room with the too-big-to-ignore-elephant of opioid addiction.

I miss Karen—her funny, sparkly nature, her outrageous stories, cleverly told and reenacted. I love her and I fear for her. Too bad I have so many vintage items around here to remind me of our auction outings. My fault, I guess, the way I always let her egg me on in bidding. And always, of course, the keepsake gift she brought me from Europe—I swear I am not making this up—an elegant little black and gold pill box.

Before she left that day, she helped me lift our little vintage desk into the back of the Subaru. It had been a present to Miles when he was about seven. That kid wanted to be an adult from the word go, I swear, and he'd been so tickled to find it tied with a big red bow on Christmas morning. All these years we'd had it parked at the beach with an embroidered tea towel over it, just waiting for the day when he'd have a child of his own. We'd now learned their baby would be a boy, and I pictured our grandson sitting at this desk, the same sort of little scholar his daddy had been.

I was not at all eager to head home. In fact, I was afraid, a confession that angered Herb when I made it over the phone to him. He saw himself as everybody's loving caretaker. That I'd claim to be afraid of him was a grave insult, plain evidence I'd lost my mind. I couldn't help it, though. I'd felt stable while on my own; it scared me what he might do or say to set me off.

But Miles and Ziwei had moved out of the Jackson Avenue bungalow and were now at their new house. August 1st was the official start day for spiffing up the bungalow to go on the market. My retreat had to end.

I'd already reminded Miles about his desk, but just before leaving, I called to let him know the approximate time I'd be coming by with it.

"Uh, Mom?" he said. "Ziwei doesn't want the desk."

"What? What do you mean?"

"She says we don't have room."

"With the new house? Come on, you have almost two thousand square feet."

"Well..." He sighed. "Also, she doesn't like old stuff."

"But…but I've been saving this for you. All this time."

"I know but, doesn't the wife get to be the one who says about the about furniture and stuff?"

Maybe in *his* house. Lucky Ziwei. Pain stabbed my cheek. I started crying.

"This just makes me feel so bad, Miles."

"Well, I'm sorry, Mom. But I've got a pregnant wife here and I'm trying to keep her happy."

"I know, I know." I was glad to see him being such a good husband. "If she doesn't like old things, does that mean she won't want your old baby clothes?"

"No, she won't."

Oh, jeez, did he have to be so instantly honest, so blunt? Couldn't he hear how hard I was taking this? We're talking about classic little romper sets made from a Vogue pattern, tiny tucks in front, one blue-checked with red piping on the collar, the other embroidered with little birds and flowers. I don't know where I ever found the time to be making these with a new baby. And now he didn't want them? This was the time for him to back pedal. This was the time to *lie*.

Instead he said, "It's not like I wore Dad's baby clothes, right?"

"Well, yeah, actually you did. We dressed you in these ratty little corduroy overalls his folks saved until you wore them out."

"Well, what can I say, Mom? The Chinese like everything to be new."

After we hung up, I curled onto the sofa. Felt like I'd been shot through the face. What could he say? *What could he say?* How about *Oh, thanks, Mom, that's so thoughtful of you.* And then to his wife,

Look honey, my mom's pretty sensitive about these baby clothes. Just say thanks, stuff them in a drawer and I promise you never have to put them on the baby. Maybe just once for a picture.

I started crying. I cried furiously for a solid hour. I couldn't see much to look forward to in grandmotherhood when clearly everything I'd instinctively do was going to be wrong.

It hit me: I was not making that baby quilt. To make that quilt would just be offering myself up for a big smack-down. One more instance of putting myself in harm's way.

Herb wasted no time pointing out that I was taking Miles's rejection of the desk and baby clothes unnecessarily hard.

Oh, no—really? I hardly needed instruction in how touchy I'd become. Apparently that's how it works when your brain's fried. But it hurt. I just longed to feel like some small fraction of my husband's energy could go into explaining to our son that his mother was in bad way and it might help if he tried to be more sensitive. Instead, Herb was always trying to school *me*.

I wasn't so out of my head though, that I'd forgotten something I've always strongly believed—that we can't change others, we can only change ourselves. I knew thought patterns stuck in the useless rut of *If only he would...*meant we should be raising the red flag of dysfunction on my own sick mind and mine alone. I didn't for one minute consider asking Herb to join me for marriage counseling.

I would go on my own.

I'd always been a big fan of the book, *Feeling Good*, by David D. Burns, M.D. Apparently considered a gold-standard classic of self help on the subject of cognitive behavioral therapy, the basic idea is to skip the psych meds and, instead, learn how to re-frame your thinking. Maybe a therapist could help me figure out how to apply this to my current situation.

I ran yet another search for local counselors. Anybody who dealt with drug withdrawal was apparently connected to a clinic where the emphasis was on attending group meetings and being monitored for relapse.

I didn't need that. I just needed to be on somebody's radar as a troubled person. I needed somebody signed up to officially be on my side. Somebody I could talk to who could help me keep these relationships of mine from circling down the drain.

On my computer screen a name I recognized popped up: Madeline Rubin. I'd met her at a Luckiamute Watershed Council meeting concerning the eradication of invasive species along the river. I remembered her as an attractive woman about my age who somehow just looked like she had it together. When we were introduced, she already knew who I was, and said she used to bring her kids out to our farm to choose Halloween pumpkins back when we were running our place as a u-pick fruit and vegetable farm. She'd read *Nekomah Creek* to her son and daughter.

I emailed her and made an appointment. I liked that she knew me as a basically sane person. I didn't want to have to spend time and money convincing a counselor of this. She and I could cut right to the chase.

I wondered what she'd think, seeing how the quirky, funny family from *Nekomah Creek* had turned into a group of people I just did not think I was going to be able to survive.

CHAPTER 15

—————————————◄

My memories of Black Butte Ranch go back to its beginnings. My parents had always admired the beautiful green meadow flashing between the pines as we drove past on our way to camp beyond Bend at Cultus Lake. A crying shame, they declared, when word got out that it would soon be developed as a resort for rich people. The initial marketing campaign did indeed target the well-to-do, including many doctors, who received the handsome flier featuring the simple and tastefully understated catch phrase: *There is a place.*

When the development was accomplished with award-winning environmental sensitivity, my mom and dad relented in their scorn. It also helped that it turned out you didn't have to be rich to rent somebody else's second home there for the weekend.

Herb and I logged good times at Black Butte during our early years together, mainly cross-country skiing with my parents, my brother and his wife. One record-breakingly cold winter the ponds froze, and Sally and I were out there on ice skates, both of us newly pregnant with the first members of the next generation.

Because of how it ended, though, my starkest memory will always be my parents' fiftieth wedding anniversary party. They'd rented a house for a week, and everyone came for a family dinner at the lodge the evening before the anniversary-day barbecue. Miles was turning a rather snarky seventeen that very day, and at some point, having endured all the family togetherness he could handle, he got up, announcing he was going back to the house.

After the dinner we drifted outside and gathered on the lawn for a family portrait. The last one my father would ever be in, as it turned out. We're all there. Except for Miles. I later thought this would make a great college entrance essay—his overwhelming regret. Turned out that was my regret, though. Not his.

After the barbecue the next day, everyone left except for my parents, me, Mary and Will, now ten, and their 14-year-old cousin, Jason. Mom and Dad had the house for the rest of the week and the kids were having too much fun riding bikes from one swimming pool to the next for me to even think of hauling them home.

I'll never forget my mother's sharp, panicked cry in the night. "Linda! Come here! He's having some kind of attack!"

She was crying, trying to give my father artificial respiration. I called 911. The two boys peeked up over their sleeping bags on the sofa, slid back down. They most definitely did not want to know what awful thing was happening. It was Mary who held the phone and tried to guide the EMTs to the house. Did a good job too. They came fast. Went right to work.

My mother and I sat on the bed in the next room, clutching each other in shock.

"They're trying too long," she said suddenly. "He doesn't want to be hooked to things. He just wants to go. We wrote up that paper."

I pushed open the door to where they were doing whatever it is they do to desperately stop somebody from dying. "My mom says he has one of those advance directives."

"Have you got it with you?"

Oh, right, number one thing on your list of things to bring to a 50th anniversary celebration—an advance directive.

"Because we have our protocol. Once we've started we can't stop."

"But he's said—he doesn't want this."

"Can you get his doctor on the phone?"

In the middle of the night? No way. So this is where we learned something important. If you want your advance directive taken seriously, you better have it tattooed right across your forehead, because somebody who loves you standing there giving people the word won't be good enough.

Now, panic at my father's attack shifted to distress at the thought of him hooked to every sort of medical device he never wanted. We'd blown it. We hadn't protected him. By the time they came out and said he was gone, we were actually relieved. He'd been in decline: his heart, his foreboding new PSA levels following earlier rounds of prostate cancer treatment.

He'd always liked to say he wanted to die by walking into some good Cascades fishing lake and not coming back. Later we would ruefully joke that he'd come pretty close, only first class, this graceful exit at Black Butte Ranch. We'd all been in the mountains together—even his only brother, my Uncle Bill, had come for the anniversary party—and Dad had made it a whole lot easier on us than if we'd had to send a search party up some twisty trail to find him.

My mother and I gave the sympathetic EMT woman the info she needed for her paperwork, the commemorative gift scrapbook lying on the coffee table between us. **Warren and Marolyn—50 Years of Love.**

I found Mary crying in the bathroom; told her Grampa had died.

"But he was nice!" she protested. "He took me fishing!"

Crushing new concept: nice people are going to die. I got her back into bed. Books tell you not to compare your twins. Kind of tough when you've got this little male/female observational experiment going on right in front of you. Will and his cousin were sleeping right through all this.

It was left to three generations of women—ages sixty-nine, forty-five, and ten—to sort it out.

When they'd taken my dad away, we phoned the final news to my brother and to my husband—*please come with the cars, gather us up and do the driving home. Be the men.*

When Herb and I decided to invest in a Black Butte house a few years later, we agreed from the beginning we would rent it out as much as we could, and go ourselves only when it was vacant. We booked a Realtor for a day in May 1999, and ended up buying the very first house we visited. It just had a good feeling about it. You walked in, sat down on the sofa facing the big stone fireplace, and did not want to get up and leave. The psychology of this fascinated me. This house was apparently well-established as one of the most popular in the rental management agency's listings. Good omen, I figured, if other people had also picked up on the welcoming feel of the place and found themselves wanting to return year after year.

We drove home and, the next night, phoned the Realtor with our offer. How's that for a quick commission?

Herb made me plead for a couple of years before he'd let me get going on the transformation I envisioned for the house, but once I got started, he was supportive. I was bogged down in trying to find a publisher for *A Heart for Any Fate,* and he could see full well how distracting and therapeutic it was for me to run around to auctions gathering a wagon wheel, a brass bed, an antique hitching post. The day I offered the top bid on a blue-painted oxen yoke, I saw it as a vote of confidence in myself. Someday I'd be telling how I'd insisted on an oxen yoke at a time when nobody else seemed to be sharing my passion for a fresh rendition of the story of the Oregon Trail.

We donated most of the existing furniture to a charity and brought in leather sofas, a Stickley coffee table and the king-sized bed we thought was excessive, but which the management people insisted renters expected. The rest of the chairs and trunks were antiques I'd collected and refurbished. We painted over the pale mauve walls with a rich tan, and hung them with Herb's 19th Century western oil paintings.

Our house sat on an acre-and-a-quarter lot over-crowded with spindly young pines. Forest fires were serious business around here; firebreaks mandatory. Yay! A project I could love! Herb got busy thinning with the chainsaw and I threw myself into limbing the remaining trees, dragging the felled ones into piles and, on the days it was allowed, torching them. One time Herb took the kids home for school after winter vacation and left me up there on my own for several days, happily managing burn piles in the snow.

When the refurbishing part of Black Butte was completed, though, I lost interest. We never managed nearly the family time up there I'd hoped, and I was ready to sell for years before Herb finally agreed the previous summer that the market, which had come to a complete standstill during the recession, had finally improved enough that we might make a break for it.

The rumored offer on our house finally came in accompanied by a letter elaborating on why it was perfect for this winsome family depicted in the enclosed photograph. Everybody blond, two little boys, a third on the way.

Cute, yes. But the offer was disappointingly low.

We had put a lot into that house, both in terms of money and my own refurbishing work, and it hadn't been the easiest compromise for me, agreeing to sell it furnished. We'd drawn up for the Realtor a list of what would be included in the sale—all the major pieces of furniture plus some perfect-for-Black Butte decorative items such as an antique engraving of the Three Sisters. I'd been picturing willingly leaving behind my collected treasures if someone came along fully appreciating my staging and backed up her enthusiasm with a full-price offer.

But now that wasn't happening. We were being low-balled.

Hadn't we already gone through this with Mary's cottage? In Eugene, our potential buyer had been a wealthy Canadian looking for a place to park his daughter while she went to grad school.

Okay, I knew that story. Just what we'd done for *our* daughter. This guy didn't want his daughter on the side of the campus where they burn sofas in the streets on football weekends; I didn't want mine there, either. Precisely why I carefully, patiently scouted out this little cottage on the *good* side, tucked in among the large, gracious homes of U of O's professors.

I stood my ground on the price until I had four men mad at me—my Realtor, who couldn't believe my stubbornness in not jumping on the only offer anybody'd had on *anything* in the current down market, and of course the rich Canadian and his agent. Number four on the list of those not thinking flattering thoughts about me was my own husband, who wanted to be shut of driving down to mow the lawn every week.

Finally I solicited outside advice from Realtor pal Clare, who laid on the line something I knew but was apparently trying to pretend I didn't. I was not going to get back the time—a whole summer's worth—I'd put into hard labor on the place. Forget the money, too.

Just let it go, she said. Don't even try factoring those things into the equation. By now I had the Canadian offering cash, no further inspections, no contingencies. I'd been so busy defending myself against these men, so busy saying *can't make me,* that I lost sight of the relief available so quickly and so close at hand.

Thanks, Clare. I signed. I Faxed. I was done.

I'd had to re-frame in my mind what it meant to come out a winner on that deal. Now, with three houses on the line, I was hoping this time around for more triumphant scenarios. I needed *something* to happen to make me feel like a worthwhile human being again.

I so wanted it to turn out that I'd been clever. I wanted to be like the hot blonde on HGTV's *Rehab Addict*—getting sweaty, bossing men around, turning a tidy profit. (Does she, actually? Well, never mind.) I wanted to chalk up some successfully executed projects, not just more stories Herb would throw back at me as evidence of how he'd indulged me and I'd gotten my way.

We countered the disappointing offer with a number only slightly lower than our original asking price. Now we were waiting for the buyers' response.

"So what's your lowest number going to be?" Herb kept pestering me.

"*Herb.* Did we agree we weren't going argue about it until we saw what they came up with? Maybe they'll accept our counter." We'd already learned the potential buyer's father, a corporate lawyer in Los Angeles, was co-signing on the house. Money didn't seem to be a problem.

"Come on, don't you want to just wrap this up?"

"Of course! But after all my work, I'd like to get rewarded. This woman likes *our* house, not whatever else is listed. And she's pregnant. With a third grandson. You think her husband and father-in-law are going to say she can't have the house she likes?"

"You don't know that's the story," Herb said. "Maybe the two guys just want to play golf and she doesn't give a rip about Black Butte."

He had me there. I *didn't* actually know the story. I was just doing my usual thing of trying to imagine likely scenarios, and the theme of pregnant daughters-in-law going to the head of the line as people to keep happy did not at the moment seem particularly far-fetched.

Here's what I wanted to hear my husband say:

You worked so hard on the place, honey, and it's just amazing how it turned out. I'll be damned if I'm gonna let some corporate lawyer in California rip you off.

Here's what he said instead:

"Promise me you aren't going dig your heels in like you did in Eugene."

Hey, I thought I'd done us good on the Eugene cottage, holding out for the best price possible. Now he was calling that incident up as a black mark against me?

Well, if he couldn't admire my ability to stand my ground, I'd have to try for points awarded for being sweet and conciliatory. I was still sick, too fragile to fight. And I tried to look at it from his stressed-out point of view too.

"I've thought about it," I told him the next day, "and I've decided one way I could be happy with a low counter offer is if we went over the list of the furniture that stays, and I took a few things off. Like the brass bed and the wagon wheel."

Nice girl points? Forget it. Herb hit the roof.

"Why would you want to go messing up the deal doing *that?*"

"Well, I just thought—if you wanted to accept a lower number—"

"I just don't understand you! Didn't we agree we wanted to get this over with?"

He was actually yelling at me. The pain in my cheek flared. I fled to the bedroom.

Crying time again.

The next day, when the new counter did indeed come back low, as we'd feared, Herb somehow thought it made perfect sense to allow me to amend the furniture list as a consolation prize for accepting it.

What the hell. He was calmly agreeing to the very suggestion that only a day earlier had earned me an instant, angry tirade. And he seemed to think all should be well that ended well.

I disagreed. I would have preferred he'd taken a deep breath and skipped the kneejerk negativity. I wished I could have skipped the crying.

I wanted him to stop feeding the beast of that reedy little voice in my head: *Look how you've become his punching bag*, it whispered. *He would never ever talk to anyone else in the world the mean way he talks to you.*

We had no sooner come to an agreement on the price we'd accept than we were arguing about how best and when to get up to Black Butte to collect whatever furnishings and décor we'd be removing prior to closing.

"There's no way I can get that oxen yoke down," Herb declared. "And anyway, you said once you didn't care if we left it there."

"What! What are you talking about? I *never* said such a thing."

I just could *not believe* this. He knew perfectly well what that oxen yoke meant to me. If he didn't, he might as well come out and admit he hadn't been listening to a word I'd said in the past fifteen years.

I couldn't stand it. Only two days home with him and I was already once again throwing clothes in a satchel and hitting the road for the beach.

Once there, I went straight down to the sand and walked the beach up to the creek. It was a beautiful day. I remember that. Sunlight shafting through sea mist makes Neskowin heaven on earth.

But it was crying time. I knew that. I wanted to stall, but sooner or later I had to go in and get it over with.

I had decided not to sleep in our usual bed these times when I came on my own. Instead, I used the little antique iron bed in the room we used to have crammed with bunks. The window faced south. I remember the sun flooding in, the room filling with light as I descended to that darkest of places.

If you think about killing yourself, you're supposed to tell people. I'd want to know if anybody I loved was feeling like this. I'd want to be there.

I didn't pray. I always figure the answers to prayers come in the form of other people, so why not just cut to the chase?

I cried and counted through the God-given people in my life.

If I killed myself now, Herb would just be mad. People who never get depressed seem to think suicide is nothing more than a selfish act of revenge.

I couldn't see calling my mother. It would just scare her. She'd be frantic, wanting to call 911 on me. Instead of her reassuring me, I'd wind up trying to reassure *her*, explain I probably wasn't genuinely suicidal. I certainly couldn't picture comfort arriving with strangers piling out of a van.

And I didn't really want to be dead. I wanted to be alive and well. I just needed to talk to somebody who would get that, sympathize with my desperation and hang onto me.

That couldn't be either of my sons. I pictured a call from me in this falling-apart state totally bewildering them, one more bit of evidence of the baffling nature of women. And there's no way they'd say the right thing. They were men. Right here in this very room as children they'd given early evidence of their Y-chromosome handicap.

All three kids had been horsing around. Suddenly Mary rushed from the room screaming. The boys had slammed her fingers in the door.

"Mommy!" she cried, tears streaming. "Oh, Mommy, why do dey do dat?"

Horrified, I saw she didn't understand it was an accident.

"Oh, come on, you guys. Tell her! Look, she thinks you did it on purpose!"

Do you think her brothers could manage this? Do you think they'd see what was needed and comfort her?

No, they could not. They were too busy arguing and blaming each other.

I was furious. They'd hurt my little girl. And here I was, left to do the scene that seems to come up so often in our lives, the one where the women try to comfort each other, and explain away the frequent inability of men to say to us the things we so badly need to hear.

"It was an accident, Honey. They didn't mean to hurt you. They would never hurt you on purpose."

Well, I could call *her* now. In fact, my daughter was so good at holding onto me that I felt I should keep her in reserve for the worst of psychological emergencies. She was a busy, stressed young person with a relationship of her own to nurture. I saw how easily I could become the needy mother, needy mother-in-law. That's not who I wanted to be.

But it was Mary who long ago gave me a gift of words I know I'll be hanging onto the rest of my life. She was about fifteen and the two of us we were at odds during that time, those years when she never looked at me without an expression of extreme loathing. We were driving past the Beanery on Second Street and we'd been arguing. All of a sudden she turned to me and delivered this:

"Mom, you know, don't you, that if anything happened to you, I would be absolutely devastated. You *know* that, right?"

I've always marveled at her young wisdom in that moment, how she was able to rise above and see that we wouldn't always be locked in this mother/daughter love/hate dance of separation. Maybe she already knew better than I that she didn't actually despise me.

Then there was my friend, Eleanor, who lived next door to the Jackson Avenue bungalow. She'd been staying in emotional touch by email. I thought of her. She'd be crushed if I did something drastic without giving her a shot at talking me out of it.

And there was my writer friend, Theresa Nelson, whom I would have gladly called on a daily basis. No matter how down I was about something, this amazing friend had a one hundred per cent record for having me laughing by the time we hung up. But Tess had lots of people to cheer up and talk down—a husband, sons, siblings galore, nieces and nephews, grandchildren, a mother in Texas she faithfully phoned every evening. Plus she was trying to finish up a book on deadline. I couldn't be bugging her. Besides, she had performed the Miracle of Cheering on me so many times, I knew her script by heart. I could play it to myself in my head without ever picking up the phone.

I thought of my friend Clara Hadjimarkos, who had sold us her nine acres of Benton County timber, planning to move to France to be with her musician daughter, then ended up staying in the mobile home on the property for a full year before leaving. She was like the wonderful treasure who came with the trees. I used to combine trips to limb the Doug firs with visits to her. She'd lived a brave and amazing life and was a great storyteller, something I'd come to recognize as an important trait for me in my closest friends. I loved that our paths had crossed in time for me to become one in her legion of friends before she died near Lyon at ninety-two. I hated knowing she was no longer in this world, and it was a good two years after she was gone before I stopped talking to her in my head every time I walked out into the woods. I framed and hung the two paintings she left us, and nailed eight of her pony shoes upward for good luck on the porch beam at the cabin. She was always eager to hear about our projects and flat-out rooted for me. Now, crying at the beach house, I felt she was there for me in sweet spirit, as if she were still living her engaging life in far off France.

Clara, I knew, would not want me killing myself.

Finally, I thought of that other sweet spirit, that little baby boy, curled up in his dark space, just as I was curled up in mine. He was new life, a fresh start, somebody I hadn't blown it with. Maybe he'd even like me. Besides, I couldn't let the story people had to tell him later on be that his grandmother hadn't waited for him, that she'd checked out before his arrival. What kind of a grandma did that?

Finally I decided I was in bad enough shape to justify calling Mary, darling Mary, who I still remember coming out of her room one time as a child and tearfully demanding audience over the stair banister.

"Look!" she sobbed, "I cried so hard and now my eyes are broken!"

That's how I felt, alone at Neskowin. Like I was broken. My eyes, my heart, my brain. Everything.

I called her. She talked me down.

Later, thanks to my daughter and Xanax, when I was calm enough to talk instead of just cry, I phoned my friend Gwen and sat on the deck, looking at the ocean as I poured out my distress over the state of my marriage. Gwen and I went back to the days when we'd met at the YMCA, both pregnant, swimming laps. We'd been through so much together, especially the difficulties of young motherhood. She let me rant for a solid hour, murmuring sympathy as a good friend does.

The instant I hung up the phone it rang again. It was Herb. He was worried about me. He'd been calling every few minutes, the whole time I was talking to Gwen.

"I don't want you to leave," he said. "I don't want this marriage to fall apart."

Magic words.

"Oh, Honey," I said, bursting into fresh tears. "That's all I need to hear."

I'd planned to stay several days, seeing as how I couldn't get back to work at Jackson Avenue until the guy refinishing the wood floors was done, but when I woke to thick fog the next morning, I changed my mind. Suddenly I didn't want to stay there all by myself. I wanted to go home to Herb, and phoned that I was on my way.

Walking into the kitchen at Wake Robin Farm, I found on the table a blue glass canning jar of flowers and a lime green post-a-note: **I'm glad you're home.** With an arrow-pierced heart.

Simple words. Good words. Precious words.

That note's still taped over my computer.

"I checked your pills," Herb said. "I know you said you weren't suicidal, but I kept thinking how stupid that would look if…well if I had to say I never even paid any attention to whether you'd driven off all upset with a great big bottle of Oxycodone."

"And you found them still there."

"Well, yeah."

I sighed. "Okay, well, I'm not doing any of this to scare you."

This seemed like a good reason to finally ditch those pills. I got a step-stool. I reached back behind the towels on the top shelf and pulled out the plastic bottle. From the compost bucket I fished a filter of coffee grounds and mashed the remaining pills into it. Somewhere I'd heard that was the way to do it. I stuffed this into a plastic bag.

"See what I'm doing here?" I said to Herb, holding it up. "I'm walking this out to the dumpster now."

At least I could do this one thing to be less of a pain around here.

CHAPTER 16

I wasn't signing on with therapist Madeline Rubin just because she'd read one of my books, but it didn't hurt a bit when I walked into her cozy office that first time and it turned out she'd made a point of reading another one, *Brides of Eden,* in the week since I'd made the appointment. She said she admired it.

Wow. Somebody saying something nice to me. I felt better already.

I told her my recent medical history—the surgery and the drug withdrawal, how I'd gone off of Oxycodone, Lexapro, and Propranolol.

"So, do you have any stories about people going off opioids?" I asked.

She shook her head. "Most of mine are dealing with antidepressants. And actually," she added, "I don't think I've ever talked to anybody who went off three major drugs at once."

Yeah? Bummer. Being unique was not helpful.

"I've also got this sinus pain that hits me every single day. It's the weirdest thing, right at three o'clock." I glanced at my watch. "Huh. That's funny." I smiled at her. "It's three-thirty and it's not hurting. I'm not kidding, this is the first day it hasn't hurt. You think it's totally psychosomatic and I'm feeling better just talking to you?" I didn't really think that was the case, but it did seem worth noting.

I concluded with explaining Herb's continual insistence that I was getting better.

"Seems like nothing but wishful thinking to me, though."

She looked thoughtful. "Can you keep a journal where you sort of rate how you feel? It might give you a way to see some progress."

"Oh, I already do these charts I've been keeping forever, writing down every pill I take. My weight, everything. I'm watching for something to call improvement—fewer ibuprofen, anything—but I'm just not seeing it."

She nodded. Scribbled something.

Well, if she didn't know about opioid withdrawal, maybe I could pick her brain for help with the regular therapy-type topics.

"What I just can't figure out," I said, "is why I'm coming through this with so much anger. I mean, I must be almost well, but I'm just …you know, like they say….mad at the world."

I was mad at the doctors. I was mad at everybody who seemed to think I should just hurry up and stop claiming to be sick already.

People who recover quickly from accidents and illnesses are seen as heroic, their stories making inspiring fodder for human interest spots on the TV news or in newspapers. The speed of their recovery seems proof of their bravery, determination, and the way they're doing everything right.

But I wasn't one of those people. I couldn't seem to get well. I was just a disappointment to everybody.

"I kind of feel like the whole world's against me," I told Madeline.

And then I *really* started talking. It took me a solid hour to download the plot points and scenes of conflict that had brought me to be sitting here in her office, fit to be tied.

I told her about the business of the rejected desk and baby clothes, how Miles had written a lovely apology email, but only several days later.

"And by then the damage was done," I said. "I was touched to get the apology, but I'd already hit bottom again. I'd already been in hell for a couple days. Things like this keep happening with Herb, too. I feel like I'm playing a game of *Chutes and Ladders* and every time I climb up a rung or two they shove me down the chute again. And I'm like: *People! Don't make me go back there again!* Because I get really down. I wouldn't say I'm exactly suicidal, but that's the level of desperation I feel, if that makes any sense."

I explained how I knew the difference. When I was thirty and deeply depressed thanks to no estrogen, I believe I *was* genuinely suicidal. I wanted to be dead. I honestly thought Herb would be better off without me. But I was the mother of a two-year-old son. You were not supposed to do that to your child. The low point of the entire horrific episode was having myself taken to the hospital for the night. Even then, though, I now realize I was a long way from actually implementing any sort of plan. My only thought was that if I were feeling this way, I should be turning myself in.

I remember at the hospital in the morning asking if I could go home.

"Well, *can* you?" the resident psychiatrist asked me right back. As in, *If we let you go are you going to try something?* That's when I realized: I'd been in the psych ward. I hadn't even noticed there were no curtain cords or metal silverware. Grimly amusing. I'm such a Good Girl, in putting myself in their hands, I had been deliberately signing up for the No Suicide Plan. Wouldn't searching for the means to do so be breaking a very important rule?

The state of my mind now was quite different. I very much did *not* want to be dead. I wanted to be alive and well and surrounded by people who wouldn't seem to find me so terribly difficult to endure.

As I laid all this out, Madeline was especially good at wincing in all the right places. *Oh, no. That's what he said, in those words? Ouch.* She seemed to get my stories, right off the bat.

I knew I was a basket case, something quite wrong with the way my mind was functioning, but her sympathetic expression seemed to confirm that at least I wasn't completely psychotic and out of touch with reality for feeling wounded by some of these recent exchanges with Miles and Herb.

"And there's something my husband does that's just driving me crazy," I said when I'd finished with everything else. "I was hoping this is the kind of thing a psychologist could help me learn how to deal with."

She leaned forward onto her knees, tensing. "What's he do?"

"Well, he pops his jaw."

She rocked back with laughter. "Oh, thank God. I was afraid you were going to tell me he was looking at pornography on the internet or something."

I grinned. "No way!" I was pleased to have it confirmed that jaw popping, in the scheme of things, was actually an incredibly tame bad habit.

And wasn't it sweet that it seemed to matter so much to her? I wondered if she couldn't quite disassociate Herb from Fun Dad Bill Hummer in *Nekomah Creek*. Confidential knowledge of this nice dad's pornography addiction could certainly ruin that children's book in retrospect!

CHAPTER 17

———————————

Just because I didn't usually drive the pick-up truck didn't mean I couldn't. I felt powerful, barreling that baby down around the curves after Tombstone Pass, belting out every song on my Bonnie Raitt iPod playlist. Herb was behind me somewhere on Highway 20 with the loaded and latched-up rental van; it was me driving a load straight out of the *The Grapes of Wrath*, the truck bed filled with wooden trunks, upended old rocking chairs strapped on top for all the world to see.

That's right, I had my stuff. I had my brass bed, I had my wagon wheel, I had my antique hitching post.

I'd made a point of not even watching as Herb and Will—who'd come up the east side from Bend to help—took the blue-painted oxen yoke down off the wall, but apparently it was no big deal. Twisting down through the fir-lined corridor, the Bitter Oxen Yoke Debate of 2013 was in the rearview mirror, just like Black Butte itself. From now on, no more letters from the rental agency suggesting Wi-Fi upgrades or additional cable channels or whatever it was future vacation renters would be expecting, something which had annoyed me greatly, having happily spent my beach vacation time as a child in a cabin without so much as a phone, never mind a TV. I could now ignore the emails discussing the latest contentious issue the Black Butte Board would be taking up. As my friend Eleanor likes to say, *Not my circus, not my monkeys!*

As I drove down along the Santiam and emerged into the valley, my beloved Marys Peak loomed in the western distance. I halfway choked up at the sight of it, the future looked so great.

But at home, I pulled the truck up the gravel drive, hurried in to use the bathroom, and never ended up helping with the unloading at all.

Instead, heading back for the front door, I veered to the sofa and crashed, falling asleep into another what I was coming to think of as "sick" dreams.

I would have stayed home the next day, flattened by withdrawal, but I had to go meet the buzz-haired, earring-wearing guy who would be repairing the shower stall at Jackson Avenue.

Ted was an artist in tile. Also, he played in a rock band.

I apologized to him for my spaciness, and explained my trouble with having been on opioids too long.

"Oh, sorry to hear that." Then, with a wistful smile, he added, "But you know, I always enjoy a Vicodin with a nice glass of wine."

"Ted! Oh, for God's sake. Don't tell me you're popping this stuff for fun! Don't you know it's *bad?* A whole lot of people on these addiction message boards got hooked just messing around like that."

Yeah, I sounded like his mother. In fact, this was pretty much the same thing I'd been saying to my own kids, that if I had to go through this, I sure hoped it would be a great example to them of why they should never think one instant of using prescription drugs recreationally.

Ted just shrugged. "I'm not worried."

I could see that. From his blissful expression, I suspected he was already dreaming of his next little Happy Hour.

By Thursday I was feeling better and gave Madeline an upbeat report. True, our own place had plunged even further into chaos, the front porch and every room of the house packed with the furniture and boxes we'd hauled home from Black Butte. On the good side, that place was history, and we had a full-priced offer on the Portland house.

The coming weekend I was scheduled to show up at a mass book signing at Bob's Beach Books, a popular independent bookstore in Lincoln City, and Herb and I were thinking we might be getting along well enough to make a short stay at Neskowin out of it. At the book signing, I would meet up with a writer friend, Randall Platt, from Washington. Randi and I had met years before at a similar Vancouver Mall event, and had recently been keeping up a steady email correspondence. She had a beach house in Rockaway, just up the coast from Neskowin, and we'd been discussing the possibility of getting together with our husbands, the four of us, for dinner.

I made another appointment with Madeline for the following week, but it seemed a bit self-indulgent. What did I need a therapist for?

Only an hour later, I got my answer. Eating dinner on our patio, Herb and I launched into what felt to me like the fight of our lives.

The opening argument involved the Jackson Avenue bungalow, and the amount of cleaning work I still saw before me. I thought we'd agreed we were through arguing, and it absolutely stunned me that here he was, one more time, still sticking up for the kids instead of me. He just didn't get it, how desperately I needed him to have my back.

Yes, I'd said they didn't have to clean, as in no dusting on the way out. I never promised to be happy with five years of deferred maintenance in any given corner, actual damage or an oven full of grease.

Only an hour before, Madeline had been deftly sorting out the dynamics of our marriage. I was the leader, she said, and always had to work to persuade Herb to go along. She said couples had different patterns, and that's just the way ours seemed to work.

Or, at the moment, didn't. Oh, it hurt, looking right across the wrought iron table to the little plaque hung around the trunk of the crabapple tree: **The roots of a family tree begin with the love of two hearts.**

Call the arborist. We had root rot.

"Every single thing we've done from the beginning has been something I had to fight for," I said. "Starting with getting married. It's not like you asked me. So are you thinking now that was a mistake? I shouldn't have even got this ball rolling?"

No comment.

Oh, Jesus.

"*Herb*, I've just been desperately hoping that what we're going through now will turn out to be the story of one more hard time we made it through together. Isn't that our story? Haven't you been happy with how everything's turned out? Thirty-nine years. Just tell me, are you glad we got married or not?"

Still, nothing.

How many times had I wished we had our fights on tape, like some couple arguing on camera to be analyzed by a marriage counselor. I was confident I had a better handle than Herb did on who raised their voice first, how the whole debate went down. Right now I somehow wished our daughter were bearing witness. Even though this is not a conversation she and her father would ever have—they talk soccer—I could hear her sounding just like I had when I'd tried to get her bratty brothers to make nice over her smashed fingers: *Oh, come on, Dad,* she'd be pleading. *She's in a bad way. You can see what she needs you to say here! She's asking for a confirmation of your marriage. Can't you at least give her that?*

No, he could not.

"How it looks to me," he finally said, "is that you've just been snowballing for thirty-nine years, getting worse and worse. You keep talking about how I make you want to leave. Maybe you should just go ahead and do it."

Oh, God, my brain. And the pain in my face. It sounded lame to claim he literally gave me headaches, but it was the truth. When I talked about wanting to leave I saw it as a warning. A cry for help. The same as when I confessed I felt like killing myself. You weren't supposed to be having suicidal ideation. If you did, you were supposed to report it to somebody who'd care.

"So that's it?" I said. "That's how you want to go on record as seeing our story?"

He hesitated. "I give and I give and I give," he said, "and it's never enough for you."

I eased back in my chair. Something cold and dispassionate came over me. I wasn't going to cry. Not right this minute anyway.

This was not about whether I could beg this man to assure me he loved me. He did. I knew he did. And furthermore, he wouldn't know what the hell to do without me. How scary for him. I'd hurt him; he wanted to hurt me back. It wasn't that he didn't know the comforting words to say; he was deliberately withholding them.

I saw that, and right then, for the first time ever, I loved him a little less.

The next day he trotted out his all-purpose apology, the one that had lost its effectiveness about ten years ago.

"Sorry for fighting with you."

Oh, please.

"You really think you can say things like that and it all goes away by saying 'sorry?' 'I give and I give and I give and it's never enough for you?'"

"I never said that!" He actually managed to sound indignant.

"Yes, you did. Those are your words. You can't just get mad and say whatever you feel like and then try to take it back. Yeah, I know you can't stand this in me, but if you say things, I'm going to remember. Especially if it's something like 'You've been getting worse for thirty-nine years.'"

I emailed Randi: **Things are BAD here. I'm coming alone.**

So many people enjoy calling themselves writers. They'll swear they've recognized this as their destiny since the fourth grade. Also, some workshop leader probably told them they'd have more success if they took themselves seriously and *called* themselves writers.

Fine. Whatever works.

But I'm the opposite. I stop thinking of myself as a writer about five minutes after I hit the print or send button. When I meet someone around town who says, "Oh, you're Linda Crew, the writer?" I have to remind myself to give the obvious answer—yeah, that's me. They're asking for purposes of identification, not wondering exactly what I'm up to *today.*

I guess this is why, since I hadn't been writing lately, the books I sat behind at Bob's Beach Books seemed written by someone else, never mind they bore my name.

I marveled at Randi's energy in brightly engaging every bookworm and writer-wannabe who came by our table. *I* certainly didn't feel worthy of dispensing enthusiastic writerly advice.

"So," she said between customers, angling herself toward me in a confidential way, "are you really going to leave this guy?"

I'd been personally updating her by email the way somebody else might have bled their life onto a blog. Randi had been happily married for decades, but to her *second* husband. The concept of divorce was not entirely foreign to her.

"Well…." This was a tough one. "I hate to think it could come to that, but it seems like I can't be around him the way I'm feeling right now. I mean, what does it say if your nearest and dearest make you want to take Xanax, but then when you're on your own, you don't have to?"

"Yeah, that doesn't sound good."

"But, see, I know my brain's not right. Things just look darker than they should. You're not supposed to make big decisions when you know you're in some kind of altered state, right? I just have to get *well.*"

In a dim, miserable way I knew this, even if at the moment I couldn't picture how on earth Herb and I could ever get back on track again.

Later, back on the deck of our beach house, Randi and I had a glass of wine and started expanding on our life stories. I explained how Herb and I had bought the beach house just after Mary and Will were born, how we'd met at Lewis & Clark College, how we'd each come far too close to spending our lives with other people, but had wised up before it was too late.

"I have this love letter from him that I keep in a special box," I told her. "He wrote it when he came to find me in Eugene after we hadn't seen each other in a couple of years. I was engaged to another guy by then, so in this letter he's beating himself up for missing his chance with me and says something like *Oh, when you started talking about what kind of life you wanted, an old house with wood floors and a porch where we'd sit and put our feet up and a garden and trees, I thought how that was exactly what I wanted too.*" I put an exaggerated lilt in my voice to deliver his summation. "*Our dreams could mesh so easily.*" I kept my eyes on the ocean horizon. "The thing is, everything he described in that letter is what happened. That's our house. We got married in the yard."

"No kidding?"

"No kidding."

"Linda," she said, "you're not leaving this guy."

I turned and smiled at her. "You're right. I'm not leaving this guy." I laughed. "I like our stories too much." And then I remembered. "At least the way I tell them."

CHAPTER 18

Collaborating with Clare on marketing our house was hardly the giddy-school-girl fun I'd been expecting. Yes, we were friends, but she was also the beautifully-attired Realtor, checking to see how it was going, finding me hot, sweaty, and foul-tempered, my mood never improved by this painful contrast. Clare held to high standards, in every detail, for any house she represented. Watching her glance around, I thought she looked skeptical. Like, was I actually going to be able to pull this off? Hey, don't ask *me* to be the one dishing up the reassurance!

As I worked, these are the words that occupied my mind. *Fun. Leisure. Recreation.* I couldn't even remember the last time I'd experienced anything remotely akin to these concepts. *Vacation?* What was that?

You're probably wondering why I didn't just hire out some of this work, right?

Well, maybe I adhere too tightly to the old adage, popular with control freaks everywhere, that if you want something done right, you have to do it yourself.

But it's true, I swear, especially when it comes to things like cleaning. You cannot just whip out your checkbook and bingo, it's done. People can be slow to return phone calls. Or they just don't show. You begin to think you could have started in on the job yourself. And paying for the work is no guarantee of professionalism. An attempt at buying ourselves out of the work of exterior window washing at the Portland house, for example, resulted in the blasting in of water through an open kitchen window all over the newly oiled cabinets.

I always felt keenly the limits of my skill set for fixing up these houses. I could be working long and hard, sure, but I was actually covering only a small proportion of what needed doing. Plumbing, wiring, roofing, flooring—all these things were beyond me. If I couldn't manage the cleaning and painting, how was this even actually my project? I ought to be doing more than just choosing the colors.

Also, in the past, these were the sort of projects I'd *enjoyed*. Even with Herb bad-vibing me through every bit of remodeling we'd ever done, I'd always taken pride and satisfaction in my work and the results. Now, I just kept slogging away, baffled as to why the endorphins usually induced by a creative project were stubbornly refusing to kick in for me this time.

And, lastly, I didn't assign myself this summer of work figuring I'd be trying to do it all as a person completely compromised. I just started in, blindly assuming any day, surely, I'd be well. Wasn't that what Herb was always telling me? That I was getting better all the time, I just didn't know it?

It was hot August by this time. The bathroom nearly did me in. Why on earth had I commissioned white tile floors on the remodeling five years before? Oh, right, because the whole thing was going to be so pretty, so vintage-looking, with a Rejuvenation Hardware medicine cabinet and light fixtures. I'd gotten completely carried away with the pleasure of seeing it done right. And face it, I didn't figure to be the one trying to maintain white tile floors with white grout.

Dismaying discovery: a person can't kneel on an artificial knee. Trying to fold myself into a working position for floor scrubbing in a tight space was awkward initially, excruciating after just a minute or two. I'd been reading a book about our country's problem with drug addiction and the author, in surveying the state of various treatment facilities, expressed indignation over one institution's policy of forcing incarcerated addicts to scrub their tile floors with old toothbrushes. Wow. So this was deemed the worst job in the world? It was exactly what I was doing day after day.

It's one thing to work hard on a job with the satisfaction of feeling you're pulling it off. To work hard and not seem to be getting anywhere is a different story. I scrubbed so hard the grout was coming out. I had to put in more. I hate white grout! I hate any color grout! Every afternoon I'd melt down and have to take half a Xanax.

I'd become fast friends with Eleanor when she moved up from San Francisco for retirement in the house next door to the bungalow. She'd been holding it as a rental for just this purpose, and coincidentally took up residence just as I started the rehab project five years before. Our first meeting, she loves to claim, involved me standing on her porch in dirty jeans, wielding a pair of loppers. "Hi! I'm your neighbor. What are we going to do about this ugly fence?" From my selfish perspective, our paths had crossed at just the right time. She'd been there for me through this past horrible year; now I didn't want to inflict my disintegrating self on her any more than necessary.

I untwisted my body from the floor and stood up to shut the bathroom window facing her house. She didn't need to hear me crying and swearing. She'd be over trying to cheer me up and really, there was nothing to be done but for me to get through this. I was trying to take Winston Churchill's advice: *When you're going through hell, keep going.*

"Here's the deal," Madeline said after hearing about my latest fight with Herb. "People say things all the time they don't mean."

"They do?"

"Well, yeah." She explained it wasn't surprising at all that Herb tried to claim he hadn't said those mean things, and that he didn't remember them. He probably didn't.

Demonstrating how this might happen, she played the part of somebody lashing out, saying horrid, hurtful things, tearing at her luxuriant blond hair to symbolize distracted craziness. Then she calmed down, saying, "What? I never said that. Well, if I did, I didn't mean it."

She said a person's mind can trick them this way.

Great. So we had *two* tricky minds here, duking it out.

"This is really hard for somebody like me to deal with," I said, "because my whole thing is that I *do* remember things people say. And people hate me for it. Like, my friend on Vicodin. I remember asking her at an antiques auction a long time ago whether the pills actually helped her with the pain. She said, 'No.' And then right away she goes, 'Well they must because I keep taking them.' Which is just....you know...that's how it is with addiction, right? And, wow— she did *not* want to be reminded of that a couple of months ago when

I was trying to explain what I'd learned about dependence and tolerance. I mean, I'm sorry, but that's what she said."

I watched Madeline scribble a note, wondered idly if she actually typed these up.

"Also," I went on, "I honestly don't say things I don't mean. I really don't. When I say I feel like killing myself or I feel like running away to Hawaii, I'm saying it like a warning. Like a report from my brain's battlefront or something. I'm never saying *I hate you* or *I'm sorry I married you*. I'm just trying to say *Hey, I'm in horrible distress here. Could you try to not make it any worse?* So when he says, *Okay, then, why don't you just go ahead and leave…..*" I trailed off, shaking my head.

"Well, when couples fight it usually goes like this," Madeline said. "If one person keeps making noises about leaving, it's not going to be long before the other one's throwing up their hands and saying, *Fine, go ahead, see if I care*. They're hurt and they've got to defend themselves, so they'll fight back. And maybe all they've got is trying to act like they don't care."

Okay, *this* was the great part about having a counselor. She had stories! She'd listened to a lot of people. Even if she didn't have any about opioid withdrawal, she'd clearly heard from plenty of people whose marriages had hit the skids. And this sincerely interested me. What did I know about other people's marriages and their fights?

Her explanation made perfect sense. My frantic irritability *had* been hurting Herb. I'd never for a moment been unaware of the fact that I had become a royal pain. It'd been easier for him to hang in there when he was being regularly commended for his caretaking skills and receiving loads of tearful, abject gratitude from the weak, pathetic patient. Dealing with a wife who looked physically well enough and yet had turned into the Bitch of the World, constantly in tears with complaints he was actually hurting more than helping... this was entirely different.

"I think he probably sees you as strong," Madeline said, "like you two can have these arguments and he figures you can stick up for yourself."

"But I'm not strong. Not now. I'm fragile. And I just can't get him to see that. I can't get him to see that if I manage to work up just the slightest bit of energy over the idea of a project, or say something positive about our marriage, the last thing I need is for him to smack me down."

"Well, you're a person who looks ahead," Madeline said. "You can't help analyzing things. It's who you are. You're trying to figure out how things are going to go and you come up with all these plans. And it sounds like Herb's just always going to have trouble getting right up to your speed. Men do. They just think differently than we do."

"Yeah." I rolled my eyes. "I've noticed that."

"And frankly, I think you'd be a challenge for any man."

Ha!

"No, no," she started backpedaling, "I didn't mean it in a bad way."

But it was okay. I was already laughing. I knew exactly what she meant.

I was thinking Herb was going to get a huge kick out of hearing it.

CHAPTER 19

I was still a very sick person. I went back to see my PCP, Dr. Miller, and told her I continued to be under periodic attack from withdrawal symptoms. Life had been incredibly stressful and I kept getting that horrendous pain in my left sinus.

"I guess I'm really just hoping you'll have some stories for me of people who'd been through this."

She hesitated. "I'm afraid by my book, anything that's going on with you eight months after stopping the opioids is probably something else."

I pressed my mouth tight. I was confident this wasn't necessarily the case, but doctors don't react well to hearing what you've learned from the internet.

"It looks to me like you've got something going on that's flaring up in reaction to all these stresses in your life."

"Well, I'm not denying everything we've been trying to do has been making it worse, but I've lived through stressful times before without all these symptoms. So, is there anything you can do to help me?"

"Not really. Not since you've made it clear you don't want to be on antidepressants."

"I just don't want one more thing I have to go off of. Everything always has so many side effects. Lexapro makes you feel flat."

"That's true," she said, not trying to pretend this wasn't a common complaint.

"I guess one good thing I have to report from going off of these meds is that I haven't had a single one of the weird sort of nightmares I used to have when I was taking Propranolol."

I told her how I used to jerk awake at the discovery of a snake in the bed, a spider dropping from the ceiling. Herb would have to calm me down, explain it was just a nightmare. One night I'd thrown myself clear out of bed in terror to escape a dead mouse, catching my big toe in the sheet and actually breaking it, the incident being all the more memorable for happening just a week before opening night of the community theatre production I was in. I needed to concentrate on my Cockney accent, not have to worry about trying to walk without a grimace.

Whenever I'd speculated over the years if this was about Propranolol—weird dreams *were* one of the listed side effects—Herb always insisted I'd been freaking us awake forever, but wasn't the fact I hadn't had one of these episodes since going off this drug pretty good proof of my theory?

Dr. Miller picked up her pad and scribbled a name. "I'm going to refer you to another doctor."

"Really? You mean like a counselor? Because, like I said, I did start seeing a psychologist."

"No, she's a medical doctor. I send her the people I just don't know what to do with. And people seem to like her. She'll listen to you."

Oh. I sat back. Okay, I got it. I looked like somebody who just needed a doctor with the time to *listen*. I thought I was what doctors wanted—an engaged patient. But maybe I was being seen as one of the unpleasantly challenging types, the ones who seem overly preoccupied with all their different symptoms.

"You don't believe me that this is about the drugs, do you?"

"No, no, I believe you," she said, but without the slightest conviction. "And I have to admit it sounds like you're doing what people going off drugs are supposed to. You're not relapsing."

But no congratulatory tone here. My inability to get well in spite of my self-discipline seemed to earn me only suspicion. Unfortunately, I'd been seeing this doctor for only two or three years, years that hadn't been my best by a long shot. She knew me only as a sick person. She knew me as the patient who claimed to feel better on a slightly tweaked dose of thyroid med faster than she thought medically possible. She knew me as the rare patient who went completely manic on ten days of prednisone.

This is where I so missed the rapport I'd built up with my previous doctors who'd now retired or, in my beloved Dr. Kliewer's case, died.

When I was a teenager, this lovely man had seen no need to medicate away my tightly-wound young nature. I remember him talking me down with a twinkle, saying some people were plow horses and some were race horses. And being a race horse was perfectly fine.

During my knee surgery/no estrogen crises around the age of thirty, it was he who'd prescribed my antidepressants. In those days, though, it was understood you'd be taking them only until you recovered from your depression. The meds would help you hang on and keep putting one foot in front of the other until you recovered. Nobody talked about your brain being wired wrong and you needing to be on these drugs the rest of your life. Nobody gave you the pitch about correcting inborn chemical imbalances. You were sick but you'd get well. Dr. Kliewer prescribed a month's worth of whatever those old school antidepressants were and booked me to come back in thirty days so he could see for himself how I was doing.

"I can't promise your knee will get better," he told me, "but *you* will get better." And then he added something I took to heart that day and have never forgotten.

"Always remember, we live on hope."

And he had a right to make that claim. Imprisoned in a Japanese POW camp during World War II, he traded his last pack of cigarettes for a medical book somebody had kicking around and started studying it. From the camp he somehow managed to apply to Harvard Medical School. You can imagine how surprised they were in Cambridge when he showed up for classes the first day.

Many years after the war, he traveled back to Japan to meet and reconcile with the now elderly Japanese men who'd been his prison guards.

Dr. Kliewer was a man of kindness and wisdom, and I so wished I could have sat down for a little chat with him now.

I had a lot of respect and affection as well for my former ob-gyn, Tom Hart, whom I started seeing when I was eighteen and he, I now realize, was just launching his practice at what—thirty-four? He'd seen me through all my infertility treatments and, to his colleagues, bragged up my novel based on these experiences, *Ordinary Miracles.*

He would vouch for my basic sanity. If I thought he'd have anything to say about opioid withdrawal, I'd have phoned him in a heartbeat. But it's only been recently that doctors have been prescribing Oxycodone for young mothers recovering from C-sections. And even, horror of horrors, giving it to women who are pregnant.

It was he who had explained to me the advice given in medical school, that when a doctor hears hoof beats, he should expect horses, not zebras. To immediately go zebra hunting meant ignoring the more common causes of disease, which should be considered first.

This makes perfect sense. The trouble I'd stumbled into, it seemed to me, is that the more casual prescribing of powerful opioids hadn't been going on long enough for most doctors to understand the far-reaching ramifications in the population. They really have no idea how many months or years it takes for someone's brain to finally heal from the damages done by these drugs.

My gut told me that in my case, the narcotics were the horses. To chase after the zebras, some different, more exotic diagnosis—Chronic fatigue syndrome? Fibromyalgia? Lyme disease? —would just be putting myself through a lot of expensive tests while making myself crazy. Okay, crazier. All the while fattening my file with the negative results which would read to future physicians as glaring evidence of hypochondria.

When I got home I looked up the website of the new doctor Dr. Miller had recommended. In the list of all the most baffling syndromes she purported to treat, I saw no reference whatsoever to issues of drug withdrawal. Nevertheless, I made the call.

Before it was ever returned, though, much later, I thought of something Dr. Miller had said almost in passing as I walked out her door.

"I'm concerned about your use of Xanax, because you know, *that's* something that can really be addictive."

I got out the sheaf of my meticulous graph paper med charts to refresh my memory. I'd first been prescribed Xanax by Dr. Herrick when we went to China for our son's wedding. I was sounding nervous about traveling apparently, so that without my asking, he'd handed me the prescription along with one for Ambien.

At the time, I'd been grateful. China was heat, humidity, and culture shock. We were trying to show the flag as the American parents of the groom in a town where no one spoke English and we spoke no Chinese. *Wo bu ming bai*—the only phrase that stuck with me from our crash course in Mandarin—*I don't understand.* Every six hours I felt sufficiently stressed so as to have no trouble at all justifying another Xanax tablet. I took the entire bottle of twenty-five over ten days, which addicted me so that what I thought was my first ever experience with jet lag was actually compounded by benzo withdrawal.

This scared me off the stuff. It was not until eight months later, when I saw the neurologist I checked in with annually about my migraines, that I mentioned how effective I'd found the Xanax when taken in conjunction with my regular migraine meds. At least the anti-anxiety properties of the drug kept me from beating up on myself and exacerbating the whole thing. She said absolutely, it did help, and she'd be glad to prescribe it for this purpose. She gave me no warnings about long-term consequences. We were on friendly terms; we'd both had sons in China. It seemed I was being treated as a person who obviously didn't need to worry about becoming an addict.

Despite her casual attitude, I was leery. I'd had such a hard time coming off the Xanax after the wedding trip. Almost reluctantly, I accepted a prescription for a scant ten tablets that I planned to make last six months.

But here's the seductive thing about Xanax—it just works so well. And fast. It seemed perfectly suited to somebody like me, a middle-of-the-night worrier. A Xanax tablet at 3:00 a.m. would turn my racing mind off and allow me to fall asleep. Much gentler than the knock on the head Ambien delivered. If it gave me a good night's sleep—everyone knows how important that is—what was the harm? I was a disciplined person. I was not an addict type. Surely somebody like me could be trusted to keep this in what I thought of as my little Tool Box for Coping With Life.

Although Dr. Herrick ended up writing the continued refills for this prescription, he was not enthusiastic.

"Try not to feel so fearful about being awake in the night. Read or something."

"I know, I know."

"At least don't be taking more than two or three of these a week," he said, although he never did explain what the long term problem with benzos might be. He never mentioned existing protocols suggesting limiting the prescribing of benzos to three or four weeks, max.

I don't break rules, so I never went over his stated limit, but I noticed, looking at my charts now, that I also never failed to find a reason to take the maximum. And here was the biggest surprise: How far back in my five years of charts did my Xanax use go? All the way. Of course. Good girl me, that must have been why I started the charts in the first place. I knew I wasn't supposed to be popping these pills without paying attention.

At some point I had realized I could get the go-back-to-sleep benefit from just a half-tab—.25 mg. But instead of sticking to the letter of the doc's law in terms of limiting myself to two or three times a week, I assiduously adhered to the total dosage rule instead, inadvertently falling into a habit of actually taking Xanax more often.

I would have sworn my Xanax intake averaged just a half a tab a day, but when I looked at the last two stressful months, I had clearly increased to more like .5mg, a whole tablet.

Could I have built up a tolerance? Could some of the symptoms I'd been attributing to opioid withdrawal have more to do with benzo addiction?

"I'm quitting this stuff," I told Herb, and proceeded to detail my rationale.

He did not receive my analysis as any sort of brilliant breakthrough.

"Okay," he said reluctantly, "if that's what you want to do." And then, bright thought: "What about staying on the Xanax until we finish up with this last house?"

I must have anticipated this, judging how fast I fired back.

"I resent that," I said. "If this stuff is part of what's been giving me grief, and I've just been drugging myself to get through all this work…"

"Okay, okay." He didn't want to get me going. "So what's going to happen?"

"I don't know. I don't know how hooked I actually am. Or if I am at all."

"So what do you want from me on this?"

Three words had popped into my head a few days previously, so I had a ready answer.

"I think what I need is quiet, sustained kindness. Just....people trying to be nice to me until I can get past this place of forever being so touchy. Just kind of...get ready to hang onto me?"

He frowned. This probably seemed to him like I thought I was entitled to have every last thing my way. I honestly didn't mean that.

"Can't you be more specific?"

"Honey." I sighed. "I can look back and say stuff like I wish you hadn't made such a big deal out of the oxen yoke, but how do I know what's gonna happen next? Just....try to be *merciful*."

I usually kept in touch with my friend Lynne by email, but now I picked up the phone. I told her about my doctor visit and my new hypothesis of what might be wrong with me: I needed to get off Xanax.

"You're not going to go cold turkey, though, right?" Lynne had spent months tapering off of just a few weeks at a full dose of Klonopin, another anti-anxiety drug in the class called benzodiazepines. She sent the link for a site called BenzoBuddies, saying the people posting there had been her mainstay of support.

I was immediately struck by the difference in the posts on the BenzoBuddies board and what I'd read in all the scattered sites frequented by opioid users, abusers, and addicts trying to get clean. People here sounded more literate, their forum more tightly monitored. The posts were dated up to the minute, the suffering pouring out onto the internet in real time.

I quickly grasped Lynn's concern for me as I read the warnings against cold turkey benzo withdrawal, which can apparently produce deadly seizures. But I hadn't been on a high and continuous dose, and if Xanax was part of my problem, I couldn't stomach the idea of one more crumb.

My plan was simple. When I couldn't sleep that night, I didn't take a Xanax. And then I lay awake. I continued to lie awake. Without taking a Xanax. A lot of my friends talked about being awake at three in the morning. We joke about having a club, going on-line. So at first this wakefulness wasn't alarming.

By five in the morning, though, I was a wreck, weepy with frustration.

It's hard to say why insomnia is so miserable. On the face of it—You can't sleep? Big deal. But isn't there something about deep sleep and dreams cleaning up the poisons in your brain?

Herb gets into bed each night and sleeps; that's it. In all these years, I've witnessed maybe a half a dozen restless nights. He'd get up with the babies when necessary, but then it was right back to bed and sleep. He has absolutely no comprehension of the desperation of true insomnia.

That's no doubt why, when he got up the next morning at six, waking me from the hour of sleep I'd finally managed, he thought he was doing me a favor when he said not to worry, I could go right back to sleep. He'd be sure to wake me in time so I could be ready to get down to our appointment at the title company at nine.

I was a zombie, signing the Black Butte sale papers. I'll bet the title officer figured the unloading of this house was about the splitting of property due to divorce.

This is the kind of insomnia where you can't even sleep when you try to catch up the next day and everybody's leaving you alone to give it a shot. Only one other time in my life could I remember feeling this way: when we came home from China and I was unknowingly withdrawing from Xanax.

So, guess what? I'd been hooked again. Oh, no, excuse me. I was just physically dependent, not addicted. But, good news! My hypothesis was correct. All I had to do now was *not* take this stuff anymore. I'd finally hit on my own cure and no doubt very soon I'd be completely well again.

Herb wanted to be helpful, rustling up new sleep music or whatever, but I was too crabby and sleep deprived to play the grateful patient.

"Just sleep upstairs, okay? Then if I'm up and down all night, at least I won't be bothering you."

After reading more on-line withdrawal stories, I'd gone to bed prepared to take a small "rescue" dose, but it turned out it wasn't necessary. Amazingly, this second night, I slept. A miracle, as anyone who's suffered insomnia knows. But then, the third night was the worst.

What a perplexing horror, the inability to sleep.

I still remember my eighth-grade English teacher, Patricia Lewis, assigning us the memorization of certain lines from *The Rhyme of the Ancient Mariner*.

Oh, sleep it is a blessed thing, beloved from pole to pole.

"Each one of you," I will never forget her saying, "will come to a time in your life when something so horrible has happened, you will feel if you could only get to sleep, maybe you could get through it."

I wonder if she had any inkling of the way she had emblazoned herself on my memory, intoning these unforgettable words. I cannot be sleepless for more than an hour without thinking of Mrs. Lewis. I can see her; I can hear her voice.

I couldn't imagine what Clare thought of me as we sat in the living room of the Jackson Avenue bungalow the morning following that second completely sleepless night. I must have looked lobotomized, struggling to process her remarks about the Realtors-only open house she'd be hosting in a couple of days. I think she said breakfast quiches would be involved.

I stared at her, dully agog. She was so....*together*, spinning out these bright sentences, one after another, and looking so charming while doing it.

"Your blouse even matches the settee cushions," I pointed out.

Herb and Clare both turned and looked at me. Did I see a glance go between the two of them? Clare readjusted herself and preened gamely, promising to wear something similarly suitable on open house day.

Herb was smiling at her. "You can be the arm candy for our house."

Huh. She was the arm candy, I was just the totally out-of-it drudge who made the place look lovely enough to warrant her fancy four-page brochure.

On August 27th, the Personal Journal section of the *Wall Street Journal* ran an article about something called Time Perspective Therapy. Instead of just dredging up hurts of the past, a person was invited to determine which of six different outlooks they took toward the past, the present and the future. The healthiest profile was the one my old self used to embody: I treasured the stories of the past, enjoyed the present without going overboard in self-rewarding hedonism, and had a planned out, goal-oriented future.

Didn't this just nail it, then, why I had lost any semblance of mental health? My sense of our stories had been perilously undermined. I thought we'd been living the story of a strong, happy marriage, but now Herb had me doubting.

As for the future, when I'd shown him a newspaper picture of writer Joyce Maynard getting married a second time in a meadow with a flower wreath in her hair, hinting I might enjoy justifying a similar get-up for our fortieth anniversary party, he had one comment: "You better wait and see if we make it."

Oh, my God.

And the present? Obviously, it was absolutely unbearable.

It makes me sad, remembering how I kept trying to force my poor brain to somehow think through this. How I kept clinging to the assumption that I would be well as soon as we put this stressful real estate business behind us.

I still didn't get it. My neurotransmitters were damaged in a way that could not be fixed by any kind of cognitive therapy. I was trying to operate without the full complement of feel-good chemicals a healthy person needs. It didn't matter what I did or where I went, how many candles Herb lit or how many hours of soothing music he played. Until my brain had healed enough for me to be well, I was going to be sick.

On the sixth night after my jump from Xanax, lying in bed alone, hoping for sleep, I suffered a frightening full-torso cramp. It was the most horrific feeling ever, and I'm sure I'd have been yelling for Herb to dial 911 except...I *recognized* this—a horrid sensation I'd experienced perhaps a half-dozen times in the past few years, only this time delivered in a much more severe rendition.

I'd told no one but Herb about these incidents. My back on the left side would suddenly cramp up clear through to my chest and I'd be plunged into instant terror. This never happened when I was under any particular stress, yet somehow these attacks involved a definite component of anxiety. I always thought the weird cramping itself had scared me—too close to how you imagine a heart attack. What to do, what to do? Of course—take a Xanax! Soon I'd be okay, with that everything's-going-to-be-fine feeling calming me. So it was all in my head, right?

Now, waiting out the cramp, which eventually subsided as they always did, I wondered—could those episodes have been a tolerance-induced expression of physical anxiety, the drug saying in effect, *Hey, you haven't taken any of me in awhile. Don't you think it's time?*

Good news, in a weird way. One more side effect I wouldn't have to deal with anymore. Also, the pain in the backs of my thighs had flared up dramatically. If that had to do with benzo withdrawal as well as opioid, maybe I could look forward to a rapid diminishing of these symptoms as well.

"You went off cold turkey?" Madeline said at our next meeting. "Jesus, sometimes you scare me."

I assured her I wasn't having the sort of brain zaps she heard about from other patients going off of antidepressants. What I did notice was all the physical symptoms of anxiety occasionally overtaking me, a knotted stomach, a certain trembling. A sort of free-floating anxiety visited upon me without the slightest relation to anything stressful actually happening at the moment. This seemed akin to what I read on BenzoBuddies, how people on some benzo for years would develop a tolerance for their dose and experience episodes of *increased* anxiety.

"Now I'm not only worried about the people I know on pain meds," I told Madeline, "I'm worried about the people who mention taking Xanax to sleep. Now I can see how Lynne probably wanted to shake me when I talked about Xanax helping me in the withdrawal from Oxycodone."

And I seriously wish she had! But have you noticed this? The Golden Rule doesn't always work so well. Because we're different; we don't always want the same thing done to us. I look back and wish anybody who could have given me a stern heads-up on any of this had not been so reticent about doing so. And yet now, when I try to "do unto others," people do not necessarily want to hear about it.

I'd been remembering a lunch I'd had with an old high school classmate who'd come home for her mother's funeral several years back. Over chicken salad I'd been lamenting my concern about how often I was finding myself wanting to take a Xanax just to cope.

"Well, I've been taking it every day for years," she said. "I couldn't even live my life without it."

My God. I wonder how she's doing now. And how much of this is going on? How many people are taking meds that, if they stopped, they'd become deathly ill? And if they continue, they'll probably have to eventually up their dose, dig their pit deeper?

Why do I suspect they will *not* want to hear from me? Um, maybe because of the way my warnings to Karen on Vicodin had been so roundly rejected?

Well, for the time being, I had to mind my own business, and I had plenty to mind.

I hadn't even realized just how much of my time and emotional energy had been going into daily debates with myself over whether or not I could justify a dose of Xanax.

Don't they say that's a defining sign of addiction? Always thinking about your next fix?

Suddenly I didn't have to do that anymore. I was no longer a person who took Xanax.

"Okay," Herb said. "I'll go to Cowboy Dancing with you."

The universe hushed.

"What? *Really?*"

"Yeah, if you still want to."

Okay, this was *huge*—a moment not so much unexpected as completely not to be believed. My husband was speaking aloud words I could never, in my wildest dreams, script for him or dare imagine him delivering.

You'd think I'd remember the setting of an exchange of such import. I can recall the exact location and circumstances of just about every conversation I report in this book, including the ones that go back to my childhood. But this one eludes me. Had I been once again lamenting the fact that he *wouldn't* go dancing? Complaining about the general lack of anything even faintly resembling fun in our lives?

Beats me. I can only surmise that at this particular lowpoint of my compromised cognitive function, this huge concession on my husband's part simply overloaded my circuits, and this one astounding item of information was all my poor, sick brain could register: the stubborn cotillion truant was agreeing to take me dancing!

"So, do you still want to do it?"

Actually, right at that moment, no. In theory dancing was supposed to be fun, but I felt physically, emotionally, and mentally incapable of even considering any attempt to engage in the concept of pleasure. Learning dance steps sounded complicated. And tiring. If somebody'd said to me, "May I have this dance?" I'd have begged to sit it out.

But dimly I remembered something I was trying so hard to believe, that I wouldn't always be feeling so sick and exhausted.

I am not an idiot.

If he was finally making this offer, I was grabbing on.

"Yes," I said, to quote James Joyce. "Yes I will Yes."

"Let me tell you a story," I said to Madeline during one session. "And you tell me how it makes you react, physically. I want to test a theory."

I then related the Story of Baby Willie and the Hot Spoon. I'd had the twins parked in the kitchen in high chairs, and I was spooning warm applesauce first into one tiny rosebud mouth, then the other. At one point, I put the spoon in Willie's mouth and his eyes went big. He let out a scream of alarm and regarded me, his mother, with horror. I glanced around. Oh my God, I had inadvertently set the metal spoon near the hot stove burner. Scorched, his tender lip shriveled. I will never forget this or be able to forgive myself.

Madeline winced.

"See, even telling you this now," I said, "I get a zap of pain down the backs of my thighs. So, do you?"

She thought a moment. "No, I feel it more in my gut. Like it makes me sick."

"Really? Okay, because I thought this zaps-down-the-backs-of-the-thighs thing was a physical reaction everybody has. This is what always happens to me when I hear a story about pain. And it occurred to me the other day that it's exactly the nerve path that seems to fire up with this very specific withdrawal pain I keep complaining about."

So maybe that's just the way I'm wired. My own personal curse. The nerves in the back of my legs retain the memory of pain. And now it's as if my brain has been told a story of pain so compelling, it finds it quite literally unforgettable.

Often as I sat in Madeline's cozy office, I'd not seem to myself like a person who needed counseling; I was just a person telling stories. The Miracle of Cowboy Dancing, for one. Madeline seemed as thrilled as I was over Herb's huge turnaround. I wondered how often in her practice she got to hear about a guy who'd seemed impervious to change just stepping up and making this awesome, relationship-saving, Hail-Mary-pass of a gesture.

The Jackson Avenue bungalow was officially on the market. Next time I talked to her, I bragged, I'd probably be telling her all about the multiple offers. Life seemed stable. I wasn't freaking out.

As long as I was here, though, I might as well get some insights for dealing with another of my long running battles with Herb—his hoarding tendencies. He had long ago rendered unusable his office in an upstairs dormer room, abandoning it after packing it to the slant-ceilinged eaves with financial files, boxes of seeds which would never be planted, even a musty, moth-eaten cougar skin. Now I wanted to re-claim and re-decorate that room for our own future grandchildren. I could picture them cozily tucked into Mary's and

Will's old matching twin beds, which I had long ago ascertained would nicely fit in there under the eaves.

Madeline provided an intriguing Rx for this dilemma: kindness. People with hoarding tendencies aren't just lazy, she explained. They genuinely have more trouble than others letting things go.

Well, I don't find the decision-making processes required in sorting out any given pile of stuff particularly easy myself, but….okay.

She suggested trying to take it a little at a time, offering him choices, resisting the controlling urge to draw lines.

Since my kick-butt tactics had never been that effective—our fifteenth wedding anniversary completely ignored because I'd insisted there'd be no celebrating as long as the shed remained in disgusting disarray—I promised to take it under advisement.

I reported our bright spots: hauling a truckload of Oregon Trail memorabilia up to the Kings Valley cabin, the deep satisfaction I felt at seeing the blue oxen yoke hanging in exactly the place on the porch that had been awaiting it. And so, too, it was with all the other paintings and rustic wooden signs. They'd all merely been doing temporary assignment on the sheetrock walls at Black Butte. Now they'd come to be displayed against vintage amber paneling where they looked so right, so perfect, so at home, that every time I walked into the little cabin, I laughed with delight.

And on the westward facing porch, there were the steps as they should be, running the full width. Herb made a point of saying they looked good.

"Really, things are fine," I told Madeline, uneasily wondering if I were simply indulging myself in the safety and comfort of having somebody listen to me. Maybe I just hated to give up enjoying her funky, eclectic décor—the vintage doll houses in the waiting room, a certain little Victorian lamp table that made me suspect Madeline and I might share similar tastes in many things. "It seems silly to schedule another appointment," I finally concluded, "but I'd like to see myself make it to the next meeting just once without having one of these crashes."

Good call.

Because the two-week stretch without a wretched downer?

It wasn't going to happen.

Not for a long time.

CHAPTER 20

I woke up weepy, but it wasn't because Herb was flying to Los Angeles to check on Aunt Catherine; I was glad to be stable enough that he could go. Seemed like it was more about the immediate and multiple offers I'd been envisioning on the Jackson Avenue bungalow *not* materializing. And feeling completely overwhelmed by our whole house still being stacked with furniture and boxes of décor destined elsewhere. Blackberry vines, the fighting back of which had been my project every year since the wedding, were now actually growing across the front brick walk. If I didn't get out there with my loppers soon, they'd be choking the house like the curse of brambles around Sleeping Beauty's castle.

Still in my pajamas, I climbed the stairs to my stationary bike and started pedaling, desperate to trigger those good brain chemicals that were supposed to fight depression. I hated being acutely aware that tomorrow marked the one year anniversary of my surgery.

Appalled. This word had been coming to mind so often and so insistently recently that I finally looked it up: *horrifying, shocking, causing dismay.* Yes, that said it. I was appalled at my situation. A whole year and I was still so weirdly ill.

So just exactly how was I sick? Clearly that's what the rest of my small world wondered. But how to explain?

It seems my brain had been bludgeoned. The symptoms of intermittent pain made no sense, and the way I was just....*on edge* was baffling. I know now it was all about my brain's inability to produce its own GABA—gamma-aminobutyric acid—the "calm down" neurotransmitter. Even the tiny amounts of Xanax with which I'd intermittently dosed myself over the past five years had taught my brain it needn't concern itself with managing this process. Now that there weren't going to *be* any pharmaceuticals in the picture, my brain had to step back up to managing this on its own. It had to heal. Until then, this lack of the necessary GABA left me feeling fragile and exposed. I never knew what might set me off and send me in a downward spiral to the bleakest depression.

Our official open house at Jackson Avenue had been held the previous Sunday. I showed up near the end to spy on the proceedings from the vantage of Eleanor's porch, and Clare came over afterward with a report of an excellent turnout of the expected curious neighbors and general bungalow fans. She mentioned a couple of visitors who might be more than looky-loos, and listed certain of my friends who'd appeared, several of whom she'd met at what I'd dubbed my Best Friends 60th Birthday Party. Daughter Mary had come by with Jaci.

"But what about my mom?" I asked.

Clare thought. Shook her head. "No, she wasn't there."

I went home and called her, a bit concerned.

She picked up the phone already talking as usual, super cheery. "Say, don't you have some tomatoes out there in your garden? Could I come get some?"

"Uh, sure. But, Mom? You didn't go my open house today?"

"Oh! Oh, my gosh. I completely forgot! I'm sorry."

We chatted a bit before hanging up.

"What happened?" Herb asked.

"Well, she just spaced it."

I felt bad. Surprisingly bad. Oh-no-here-I-go-again bad. I hadn't even realized how much I'd been enjoying picturing her getting a kick out of a certain photo I'd added to the staging just for her—the two of us holding gloved hands in our Easter finery when I was a tiny girl in a frilly dress and Mary Janes.

Everybody forgets things. A mentally healthy person understands the value in being forgiving, but my mind these days could only brood, engage in an endless loop of what Madeline called spin-cycle thinking. My mother had managed the hour drive to my brother's book-signing party on a day of record summer rains just the previous Wednesday. Then she'd driven an hour north to a friend's funeral, and another day joined fellow donors on a bus ride to a fundraising dinner at a country estate. True, she wasn't up to her usual Saturday morning breakfast with her friends, but she'd managed to phone to let them know. She hadn't spaced it.

And yet she'd forgotten me. It seemed so clear: I just wasn't on her radar.

I was still peddling when I heard Herb out at the truck. Was he leaving? I let myself down off the bike and went to my dormer office where I opened the window overlooking the driveway.

"Are you taking off?" I called.

"Apparently not. Truck won't start." He said he'd already ruled out the airport shuttle or renting a car, that he'd give himself ten minutes to see if he could get the truck going.

"Maybe I better drive you up there."

"Well, let me see what I can do here first."

I got back on the bike, but then I realized: whatever he decided to do, it would likely involve me, and that would be me not in pajamas. I went downstairs and got dressed. I put my oatmeal on the stove.

"Sorry," he came in saying, "but I guess I better take you up on your offer."

"No problem." I was thinking how Madeline said Herb seemed to have a hard time with the way my brain wanted to jump ahead in anticipation of what lay ahead. At least this time, my brain was on the right track. Because I was already a few minutes ahead on getting it together.

Make lemonade. If I was going to be in Portland, maybe I could manage a visit to my cousin Heidi. I'd been promising her a huge photo my father had taken that had been hanging at Black Butte—her grandfather (my uncle) fly fishing on some Alaskan river. I went and pulled it out of one of the upstairs bedrooms, hauled it out to the Subaru. I printed out a map of directions to her house and tossed the chopped walnuts and home-grown boysenberries into the bubbling oatmeal.

I quickly did my makeup, noticing how this little shot of adrenalin had perked me up. Maybe being needed was a good cure for depression. Plus, it would be nice to see Heidi and her new baby boy.

The timer dinged in the kitchen and I started spooning out the mush into a bowl.

Herb came in. "Are you ready?"

"Yup. Just have to chow this down."

When I told this story to Madeline two days later, I had a hard time with what came next. Because Herb didn't actually say anything I could quote.

What he did was raise his arms and drop them in a full-body expression of total disgust. A huffing out of angry air, a casting of eyes to heaven.

He was mad at me? I was hustling around to help him out and he was mad?

Great. Thank you so much. Because I knew what was going to happen now. I started eating as fast as I could. Crying.

"There! Am I shoveling it down fast enough for you?"

We got in the car. Down, down my brain sank to that black place. I leaned my head against the window and wept. What was the use of trying? I was married to a man who could not deliver the simplest of Rxs: *Be kind.*

"Should I just be turning around and heading home?" he said as we crossed the Santiam River on I-5.

"What's the use of that?"

"Well, you're not really looking like somebody who ought to be left alone."

Yeah, so? Being alone was better than being with him.

"Go see your aunt." *Go be a hero for her.*

If we said anything else the rest of the hour-and-a-half drive, I don't remember it. When we pulled up to the drop-off curb at the airport, I was struck by all the people hugging goodbye. I guess they loved each other.

I got out of the passenger seat, went around and dropped into the driver's seat. As soon as Herb had his bag out, I pulled away without a word.

I couldn't believe myself. Everybody knows you're supposed to imagine what would happen if the plane went down and this was the last thing you'd said—or in this case not said—to the person you supposedly loved. And more than most people, I'm guessing, I usually do. My mind is forever flashing with stories of what might happen ahead.

But maybe today *I* was the one with the riskier hold on life. What if *I* died? I felt cold and frozen, down here in the dark. Let them all worry about the last thing they'd said to *me*.

The return of the stabbing pain in my face told me I would not be going to Heidi's after all. Driving back down I-5, I fantasized stopping at the Jackson Avenue bungalow and yanking up the For Sale sign. I would go out to Wake Robin Farm and throw a few of my things in boxes. Wouldn't that be something if I were all moved in at Jackson Avenue by the time Herb got home?

Wait, though. That wouldn't be nice to Clare. And we didn't own the house outright. I'd still have to make mortgage payments. And pay property taxes. I'd have to sit down with this husband I didn't want to be in the same room with and sort it all out....

See? How pathetic! Even when my brain's full of gunk and not firing on all pistons it's still *my* brain, which means I can't even cook up a decent little fantasy without jumping ahead to envisioning the consequences that would spoil everything.

As I passed the Woodburn outlet mall, I impulsively turned off the freeway, parked and, on automatic pilot, headed straight for the maternity store.

When Ziwei had first arrived in the U.S., I'd taken her to have her wedding gown fitted and to shop for what I thought of as her New Life in America Wardrobe. I had always treasured the memory of the way she'd insisted on tucking her arm through mine Chinese-style as we strolled Bridgeport Village in Lake Oswego, and every time I'd passed a maternity store in the six years since, I'd dreamed of a repeat of that lovely day, only we'd be shopping for smocks and jeans with stretch panels. I certainly never pictured the conflagration of illness and real estate craziness that would eclipse the planning of such an excursion.

So now, maybe I'd risk picking out some things for her myself. At least I'd be able to say they came from one of the stores in the mall which she, like every other Chinese person, local or tourist, favors for the bargains.

I chatted with the salesgirl. She would never have guessed what a demented brain she had in her store. I chose a top, carefully avoiding the sort of thing *I* would have worn while pregnant, taking the girl's advice about the latest styles.

If Ziwei didn't want the baby clothes I'd saved, I hoped I'd at least be allowed to buy some new ones. I hit the Osh Kosh store where I found a little set of overalls and plaid shirt, the very sort of get-up we'd dressed Miles in. Size 6 months. It could be the baby's wear-to-Wake-Robin-Farm-next-summer outfit.

Heading into Corvallis, I did not stop at the bungalow. I went straight home to my computer and typed a message to Madeline. **Any chance of coming in sooner than planned? Tomorrow's the one year anniversary of my surgery, Herb's gone to L.A., and I am not doing so hot.** As I knew I would have to, I went into the bedroom, lay down and started crying. Hard. I was sick of this, so terribly weary of having my mind in this awful place. Thus the shopping-trip detour to stall the dreaded inevitable.

Eleanor, knowing Herb would be out of town, had booked me that evening for what she was calling a celebration dinner. I most definitely did not want to go, and I would have canceled. But here's the thing about this particular friend—all through this she'd made it clear I was welcome at her house whether I felt capable of being "on" or not. She *wanted* to see me, regardless of my condition. If I canceled, she'd be disappointed, and not just because she'd been looking forward to eating in a restaurant.

Also, I had to go into town to deal with the irrigation hoses at the bungalow anyway. These first days on the market were crucial, Clare felt, and everything had to be perfect. No hoses over the driveway during the daylight. Herb had instructed me exactly how he wanted the hoses rolled out for the automatic sprinkling system and how to put them away in the morning.

So, I didn't cancel on Eleanor. I went. She said we were celebrating my completion of the bungalow and my getting well. But I was not well and, sitting there having a glass of wine on the deck at Big River, I thought the main thing I had to celebrate was having a friend like her to keep me from blowing away.

I felt no better the next day. More crying, the house all to myself. And a new symptom—my stomach felt wretched. That twisted up feeling you get when you're incredibly anxious, the sort of feeling I knew could be quelled with Xanax. Oh, man, I wanted to take one. I wanted relief.

You could even use the word crave.

Maybe I'd never felt tempted to take Oxycodone after I'd quit because the withdrawal symptoms seemed so unrelated to the drug itself. I'd only been taking it for pure, massive pain. I never got anywhere near high; I had no memory of pleasure to chase in hopes of a repeat.

But Xanax—this was different. You feel anxious, you take a Xanax, very soon you don't feel anxious. You know deep in your heart everything will be all right.

Yes, I very much did want to experience that sort of calm again.

I jumped in the car and made a beeline for the bakery and a whopping loaf of Apple Crunch Cinnamon Bread. Came home, ate a big buttered chunk.

Didn't help.

I was pretty sure that throughout this whole ordeal, I'd never felt worse.

I started rationalizing. Justifying. Maybe my Xanax addiction wasn't as big of a deal as with the Oxycodone. I hadn't even been taking that much.

One pill probably wouldn't hurt.

I got up from the bed, rummaged through the medicine cabinet and found the orange plastic bottle I'd put aside two and a half weeks ago. I knocked out a tablet and swallowed it with a palmful of water from my sink faucet.

Then I lay back down and phoned Mary, catching her on her lunch hour, confessing I'd hit rock bottom again. She proceeded to do for me what she does so well, just keeping up that verbal connection. A person can't do anything too crazy if somebody who loves you is right there willing to put the time into talking you down.

Between her and the Xanax, it didn't take long.

After awhile I realized I felt well enough to take Miles and Ziwei up on their offer to have me over for dinner. I wondered if Herb had instructed them to look out for me. If so, fine. I didn't care where the comfort came from, as long as it came.

Sitting at the dining table in their new Willamette Landing home, I was grateful to be fortified by the Xanax when Miles started lecturing me on how "deeply weird" I was to have spoken with a young Chinese woman in their neighborhood. Those were his exact words. *Deeply weird.* On a bike ride a couple of months back I'd seen her in her backyard with two little boys. Mea culpa! I stopped and, over the low fence, struck up a conversation. Yes, I'm guilty of talking to strangers. Take me out and shoot me. She was friendly and seemed interested to hear that my Chinese daughter-in-law was soon moving into the house across the street, same model as hers, and would be having a baby. Ziwei was going to need some women friends. Other mothers. I'm not sure why Miles considered this practically criminal. I didn't pass any vital information; I didn't arrange any play dates. I just saw it as a possible friendship heads-up.

Thank you, Xanax. Instead of dissolving into tears, I staunchly defended my out-going nature to Miles. And then, almost in defiance, I went down to the first tribal belly dance class of the season and chatted up a cute Chinese girl in a coin belt. She was open and friendly and I told her I couldn't help it, I was always interested in the stories of Asian girls because I had a Chinese daughter-in-law. Of course I loved it when she sweetly insisted I couldn't possibly be old enough to have a daughter-in-law.

Gathering in a circle on the dance floor, our astonishingly vibrant teacher, Antigone Cook, reminded us that this was our time to forget our cares, our jobs, our families and just dance. Let loose and enjoy being ourselves. In my long velvet skirt I faced the mirrors with this wonderful group of women, none of whom knew my story. The endorphin rush was fantastic.

Deeply weird, my pretty little foot!

CHAPTER 21

I sat in Madeline's office, bemoaning the lack of the instant offer on the Jackson Avenue bungalow I'd hoped would be my big emotional fix. Daily stops to freshen the cut flowers and snag individual stray leaves in the yard were becoming discouraging, especially with no evidence of any requested showings.

Tilting her head thoughtfully, Madeline tossed out this innocent question:

"Have you considered hanging onto the bungalow as a writing studio?"

After a stunned beat, I started stammering out objections. Even if I could see myself writing again, I had a perfectly good office. I never felt like I needed to leave home to write. Couldn't picture working in a coffee shop or doing the back-of-the-bookstore, writer-in-residence thing.

"But you seemed to like coming into town and going to the bungalow. You know, when you talked about the summer you fixed it up the first time. I just thought, if you could swing it financially, maybe you'd enjoy it."

Her question stuck with me way beyond our session, knocked the breath out of me every time I thought of it because, actually, *yes*, I wanted that. Longed for it. Not necessarily to turn the bungalow into a studio, but simply to be a working writer entitled to consider how I might best arrange my creative work space.

And she could actually see me this way? Imagine this as my future? I ached with what I knew: my brain was permanently damaged. I was never going to be writing again.

The fact that the horrible anniversary of my surgery had been so gloriously salvaged by one tiny Xanax tablet had made this "rescue dose" strategy seem reasonable, but when a fresh and stronger wave of withdrawal symptoms slammed me down again a few days later, I saw that it wasn't.

But I'd learned something: I was addicted. If you have a constellation of physical and mental symptoms and the taking of one dose of a certain drug completely, if temporarily, eliminates them, however briefly, well then, you're addicted to that drug.

I swore to myself that I had already taken the very last Xanax tablet for the rest of my life.

In the world of real estate, the Jackson Avenue bungalow had not been on the market any time at all; it just seemed like it to somebody who'd watched far too many exaggerated-for-drama HGTV shows, somebody who was absolutely desperate for closure.

Following the fairytale rule of threes, the third couple to take a look—empty nesters—fell in love with my darling little cottage and made an offer. It was low. We countered.

I'll never know if this bit of the story was leaked to us intentionally or not, but the instant I heard the wife's name was Mary and that she was absolutely in love with every last detail of the house, actually lobbying her husband to come up with a better offer, any seller-buyer adversarial notions evaporated in me. I was on *her* side. This woman loves my house? Hey, let's see what we can do to help her buy it!

Clare was surprised how fast I said, "Sold!" when she told me their new offer. I'm sure she hadn't forgotten how I'd dug in on the Eugene property.

"If she loves the place," I said, "that's good enough for me."

We signed the papers on October 1st, and it would close two days later.

Finally. All three properties sold. Stress be gone! Time to start doing things I'd put off for so long, like catch-up lunches with friends. When I set up the date with my Portland writer friend Pamela Smith Hill, I commented that we hadn't met for lunch in a year-and-a-half.

Pam insisted we'd lunched at our halfway meeting place in wine country, the Dundee Bistro, in the fall just a year ago.

Certain she was wrong, I checked my emails. Oh, my God, I'd completely blanked it out. I'd gone flying up there *the very day before my surgery.*

This wasn't the first evidence of my brain sputtering in the past year. A woman said she'd seen me at the gym with my mother in the spring. I said I hadn't been there, only later remembering my mother had insisted on me trying her warm-pool exercise class. In another disconcerting episode, I went searching for my second-best watch, finally remembering I'd dropped it off for repair six weeks earlier and simply forgotten about returning to collect it.

The mind-boggling part about Pam's correction of my memory, however, was the stunning reminder that I had once been a woman who'd think nothing of jumping in the car and driving off for lunch the very day before a major surgery. And who was that person who optimistically wrote an email describing looking forward to being past the surgery so she could know that each day she would be improving?

Breezing off to lunch, that poor girl who used to be me had no idea it would be the last normal day before the gates of hell would open up and swallow her whole.

And now, here we were again, in Dundee. Over lunch with wine, I ranted over all the recent dramas. It was shocking, really, how much pent-up anger I still needed to spew.

When I finally shut up, Pam said, "I wonder if maybe you and Herb should consider separating for awhile."

My mouth fell open. "Seriously?"

"Well, I've known people who did this and when they got back together, they were quite happy. I hope it doesn't shock you for me to say this."

Well, I *was* shocked, but mainly in recognition of my own vehemence. My descriptions of our fights had clearly been leaving out something critical—my deep down, rock-solid belief that Herb was my true love and that's all there was to it.

"No, that's okay," I said. "You had to listen to all this. You've got a right to an opinion." God knows I'd delivered plenty of analysis and suggestions on *her* life.

"I just think it's too bad," she said, "that you've sold the bungalow. Because that would have been so easy for you to move in there for awhile."

"Oh, believe me, I thought about it, but no, it's a *good* thing we've sold it. I don't need that cute little house sitting there tempting me with fantasies of running away. Besides, I sort of did that during the summer when I kept taking off to the beach by myself."

Pam looked skeptical. "You two just seem like you have so many things unresolved."

"But we wouldn't dream of separating now. Not after we've just finished living through all this crap and we're still together. Things are just about to start getting good again. Hey, we're going to be grandparents! And I told you he agreed to go to Cowboy Dancing, right? It starts tonight!"

Driving home through the autumn gold hills, I thought about Pam's observation that Herb and I had issues unresolved.

As if, between two people, everything ever *could* be resolved. As I saw it, when we got married we resolved to stick together for life. Everything after that was just muddling through. We never did resolve one of the big conflicts of our early married life—the fact that even though Herb was the best hands-on dad I knew, especially in the winter, I still never had as much child-free time for writing as I needed. So we argued about this periodically, never resolving anything.

Meanwhile, the kids grew up. And we were still together. That's how some problems work. You just live through them. Live through them without getting a divorce.

The first week of Cowboy Dancing had been something of a bust. The only other people signed up besides us were two single women. Ernie, the instructor, said no problem, we would trade Herb around.

"Hey, sorry," I said. "I don't feel like sharing him."

I felt bad for these women. Like me, they wanted to dance with a man. But look what I'd gone through to get mine here! If you showed up at a marriage rescue retreat and heard you'd be lending your husband out because a few others hadn't made it, would that be just fine?

I don't think so.

Ernie was nice about it. He said actually, if they couldn't round up more people, this section of the class couldn't go anyway. Then he started showing us the two-step.

I'd promised Herb fun. A room full of dancing couples. This vision hadn't materialized, and I was willing to concede. He'd made the effort. Points to him for that. I'd give him a break and we'd get our money back.

But something interesting was happening. Herb wasn't hating it as much as he'd feared.

Walking out, he said, "So, do you want to go over to the other class in Albany he talked about?"

"Seriously? I wasn't going to make you. You really want to?"

"Well, yeah."

Wow. Go figure.

He gave me his sweet little smile. "I guess I liked seeing you get all lit up. I like the idea of seeing you get what you want."

Okay, I remember the mean things people say to me, but I remember the good things too. I wouldn't be forgetting this!

So tonight we'd head over to the Albany campus to join the larger, already established class.

I was excited. That afternoon I already had on my long denim skirt, and I was sashaying around town doing errands, taking a pie to the people who'd bought the house, meeting them for the first time.

Standing in the house that now belonged to this Mary Nelson, admiring how nicely her Stickley furniture echoed the craftsmen style of the house, hearing how much she loved every last design detail…well, it was absolutely intoxicating. She was giving me something I'd missed on my other projects without even realizing it—pure appreciation for what I'd accomplished from the person who was going to live in the house and enjoy it.

My kids had always been glad enough to have landlord parents giving them leave to promptly call in repairmen as needed, but I have no memories of any of the three of them raving in delight at their new digs as they moved in. No gushing. No *Oh, Mom, I just LOVE these cabinets!*

Well, really, do anybody's kids talk to them like that?

Still, to have this woman unabashedly in love with the house was quite simply the purest affirmation I'd had in ages.

At least a dozen couples milled around the mirrored room in the community college's gym building. This was more like it! The women all had their own men. Guess I was the only one quite so excited, though, wearing a skirt like I was going to a party. Ernie, the teacher, welcomed us. He helped out on this class with the official instructor, Vickie.

Fresh start on the Two-Step. Slow…slow….quick-quick…slow…slow….quick-quick.

Just a few minutes into it I had to shrug Herb's right hand off my shoulder. "Your hand's supposed to be under my arm on my back."

He dropped his arms and stepped back. "Okay, here's where we're going to have trouble. You aren't going to want to let me lead."

Uh-oh.

I winced. "I'm not allowed to say you've got your hand in the wrong place?"

What happened to *I just like seeing you all lit up?* He'd lashed out with this failure-to-follow gripe so fast, I could only think he'd had it at the ready, having heard this repeated by touchy men before him. Women could be like this, everybody knew, and certainly I must fall on the bossy end of the spectrum. Naturally I'd refuse to follow. He'd been expecting it.

Nervously I rearranged myself in his arms and we started again. I smiled at him. We were doing okay. We liked country music. This was fun. I couldn't believe it. I was actually dancing with my own sweet husband. I'd been longing for this forever. I'd been convinced we were doomed to grow old and die before ever spinning around a dance floor together.

I'm afraid I was exhibiting more enthusiasm than coordination at this point, though, and my stumbling steps seemed to frustrate him. Maybe my brain still wasn't working quite right? Maybe I'd do better when I was completely well?

Standing there, winded, as the instructors positioned themselves to demonstrate some new turn, I tilted my head toward Herb and whispered, "This is so great, I'm having fun even though you're mad at me!" And I meant that. I could see he was annoyed, but for the moment I was just so damned thrilled, it seemed to override everything else.

Toward the end of the class, though, he really lost it. He stopped in his tracks, backed away, lifting his arms, turning a fed-up sort of circle.

"What?" I said, dismayed. "What did I do?"

I felt the instructors eyeing us. Embarrassed, I wanted to fall through the floor. Surely Herb's impatient body language had been broad enough to be noticed by every single person in the room.

Ernie came over and danced with me. Vickie danced with Herb.

So, yes, we obviously needed breaking up.

At the end of class, Ernie gave a little talk about how this could be kind of like date night. How we had to be patient with each other. He was glancing at Herb, glancing at me. It was not my imagination. We were the problem kids.

I said nothing as I trudged beside Herb out to the car.

"Kind of weird how we did so well last week and then didn't tonight," he observed as he pulled out of the parking lot.

Seriously? No mystery to me it seemed that way to him. Last week he'd been the only guy, a hot property. He could do no wrong. Tonight a dozen other men in jeans and boots totally had it together. They didn't have to complain their wives wouldn't follow. They knew how to lead.

"Why did you *do* that?" I said at last, sensing the protective endorphins draining away.

"Do what?"

"Do *what?* You humiliated me. You were mean to me in front of all those people."

"Sorry. But you kept getting the step wrong."

Oh, Jesus. He was never going to get it. Mean is mean. Guys who actually hit their wives always have some stupid explanation too. She asked for it. Ticked him off. Made him mad. I wouldn't bother trying to draw this parallel again, though. Herb Crew, sainted husband and father, would brook no insulting hint of either his words or behavior ever edging one inch over the line into being categorized as abusive.

I tilted my head against the cold window glass all the way home, saying nothing. My brain felt raw, exposed to the hurt. I was drifting down into that black hole again. Only hours before, with several good days in a row behind me, I'd dared to hope I wouldn't have to spend one more hour in that hellish state.

Tricked again.

My stomach was churning exactly the way it had when he'd gone to California and I'd resorted to a Xanax to stop it. At home, I walked in and put on the kettle. I got out a stack of bills and, robot-like, sat down in the breakfast booth to pay them as I drank cup after cup of peppermint tea, trying to stop the horrible feeling in my gut. I was stalling again, dreading what I knew was coming.

Herb turned on the music and came into the kitchen, holding up his arms.

"I guess we ought to practice like Ernie said."

I stared at him. Practice dancing? What for? I couldn't show my face in that class in front of those people ever again. He just didn't get this at all. He didn't understand the damage done. Thanks to him I was back in the pit. Pretty soon I knew I'd be wondering again if it really was worth trying to stay alive.

Again I cried long and hard while Herb watched recorded soccer on the other side of the house. I believed him when he later said he never heard me. And I didn't care. He couldn't help me. He was the one who'd shoved me down here in the first place.

Pain stabbed me awake in the middle of the night. Felt like a knife in my gut. Xanax would fix this. I *needed* it. But if the Xanax had fixed my gut ache so fast and efficiently last time, didn't that probably mean that the intensity of this knotted stomach was itself a withdrawal symptom? Maybe I wasn't just feeling crushed about the dancing. Maybe this was Xanax saying *Take me! You know you want to. You know I'll have you feeling like everything's gonna be okay in no time flat!*

I finally went back to sleep again, but it seemed pretty clear:

I was never, ever going to get well.

I felt no better in the morning. And I was supposed to go out to lunch with my mother. Well, I just couldn't. My brain hurt. That's how I'd come to think of it. Not like a headache. My brain hurt the way your heart hurts when it's broken.

I stalled on calling her, hoping for a miracle of recovery, dreading her annoyance, plagued by recall of one her favorite mantras: "Don't you just hate it when people can't be enthusiastic when you ask them to do something? Don't you just hate it when somebody wimps out at the last minute?" When I'd replied so promptly and cheerfully to her invitation a few days back, she'd laid the positive reinforcement on to a degree terrifying in retrospect, now that there was no way I could come through with the upbeat behavior of which she so heartily approved.

I was sniffling when I finally called her. "I'm sorry, Mom. I just can't make lunch. I'm feeling really bad again."

Long pause. "But you sounded so good the other day."

"I know, but I guess that's how this thing goes."

She sighed. "Well, I'll just have to move on to Plan B. I don't suppose there's anything I can say or do to make it better?"

"Um…just don't be mad at me?"

"I'd never be mad at you for something like this."

That night she phoned again to see how I was doing. I took the phone to the bedroom, dropped to the antique love seat and tried to explain. I told her how I'd come crashing down the night before when Herb was so rude to me at Cowboy Dancing.

"Well, that's not drugs," she said. "That's just a bad husband!"

"But Mom, it's the way the drugs have messed up my brain. Because yeah, he wasn't nice, but I can see that something's going on that makes me take everything so much harder. I know he's doing his best to drag me through this, so I'm not going to blame it all on him. Don't you realize what a big deal it is that he agreed to go to that class with me in the first place?"

"Well, yes, that's very nice of him."

"And the thing is, Mom, I crashed pretty much the same way when you missed my open house."

Well. Clearly this was entirely different.

Her voice went cold. "You don't know everything I had going on that week."

"Yes, I do, because you told me. But that's not the point. I'm just trying to say that I know my brain's not right and I don't want to be blaming everybody else because I can see this is *my* problem." I started crying again. "This whole thing has just been so awful. And I've just felt so alone."

"You're not alone. You've got Herb."

I focused on the brass bed I'd spent a good part of the day lying and crying on.

"Sometimes, though, it seems like he's just the one making everything worse."

Ignoring this, crying now too, she said, "You don't even know what it really means to be alone. And I just can't imagine how you'll do when you're eighty-six and you don't have Herb."

Oh, my God. Had she really *said* this? I thought we'd long ago agreed we were not the sort of family where people say the worst things they can think of to each other. I thought we all understood the rule about not saying things you couldn't take back.

"And you know," she continued, "what I'm always wondering is—*where is your gratitude?*"

My heart was pounding; I was shaking. "Mom? I'm hanging up now."

And for the first time in my life, that's what I did.

I rushed out to the kitchen where Herb stood at the sink.

"My *mother*," I screamed, and slammed the phone to the floor.

"Whoa." Eyes wide, he pulled back. Then, watching me warily, he stooped to gather the popped-out, rolling batteries.

Later he confessed his relief that at least I hadn't been aiming at him.

I cried for quite awhile after that, but in the morning I woke with a strange sense of relief.

My mother was never going to understand this.

It was time I gave myself permission to give up trying to make her.

CHAPTER 22

Just don't be mad at me.

This became my stock answer when Herb would ask if there was anything he could do or say to help. No magic words could make me well, but I had definitely figured out the sort of thing that could send me spiraling downward.

I couldn't bear to have people annoyed or impatient with me, couldn't stand any hint people suspected I wasn't handling whatever weird problem I had in the proper way. Bad enough to feel so horrid without also being under suspicion. How could I be claiming to be sick now when last week I looked just fine?

If nobody else understood me, at least the internet knew perfectly well what was up. I was obviously a desperate drug addict. Pop-up ads continually invited me to reach for the help awaiting me at one lovely spa-type rehab facility or another.

I would click and devour the ad copy, soaking up words like compassion, comfort, caring, help, sensitivity, healing.

One place was actually located in the gorgeous old Hollywood neighborhood of Hancock Park. I fondly remembered walking those leafy blocks with my friend Tess as she pointed out houses where movie scenes had been filmed.

What if I checked in there? I could see Tess. It would be lovely.

But then I'd remember. These facilities were for people who needed to be forced off their drugs. They would be locked in. Their urine would be monitored. It was all about compliance. And when they got out, ostensibly "clean," they'd still have to live through the protracted withdrawal symptoms, do the part I was trying to get through now.

Nobody ever seemed to have the answer to the big question that mystified me: once you're clean, how long until you feel well again? Apparently, given the appallingly high rate of relapse, this was a question rarely ever raised, much less answered.

Seek medical advice warned all the websites.

And good luck with that.

Finally, during one of my desperate, middle-of-the-night searches, up popped a doctor in my own town who had started a clinic specializing in addiction. Susan Spaulding. Must be new. Surely I'd have seen her listing in all the previous times I'd Googled "drug addiction withdrawal doctors."

In phoning, I feared I was in for some square-peg-in-a-round-hole arguing, because this was apparently a clinic dispensing Suboxone, a drug something akin to Methadone, for people trying to get off of opioids. I had no intention of complying with their process of vetting for this prescription. All I wanted was to talk to somebody who had some expertise in this area, somebody who could tell me some stories.

My call went directly to a recording, a cold voice completely belying the warm fuzziness of the clinic's name. I was directed to leave a message, then wearily admonished to *please* (you could almost hear the *for God's sake*) not leave repeated messages.

Rebuffed, I hung up. It's not like this was an easy call for me to make. How much harder would it be for addicts bearing far more baggage than I? Didn't these clinics *want* people to get help?

"Maybe most of their clients are there by court order," Herb suggested. "They're not set up for somebody like you."

"Yeah. Got that."

I took a deep breath, picked up the phone, called again and this time left my message.

I needed this woman's knowledge.

I've always prided myself on my decisiveness. One of the biggest, most life-altering choices I'd ever made was to break off with the guy I was engaged to my senior year of college. I'd been all set to follow him wherever he was accepted to grad school, but he seemed to be getting cold feet and, like a little kid, acting out on it. While his parents saw me as the bad girl who'd led him astray—laughable to me, Goody Two Shoes—he started messing with a married girl. *Married.* I was *so* not interested in hearing about how she didn't really *consider* herself married or whatever idiot way he was spinning this. I'd been warning him that if I decided to call it quits, that would be it. I wasn't going to be one of those girls who go back and forth, dragging out the drama. I hauled him into one of the campus counselors, figuring he needed schooling in just how badly he'd been treating me. Instead, after hearing the lowdown, the counselor turned to me and said, basically, this is how he is. Can you live with it? The decision is yours.

Well, no, since she put it that way, I couldn't. I wouldn't. I deserved better. I broke up with him between her office and the dorm elevator. And I never looked back, not even when he claimed to be surprised at how firmly I was holding to my decision and begged me to reconsider.

Because of the way this decision had, in short order, led to the bliss of reunion with Herb, I became a big believer in extricating myself from situations that were going to wind up hurting me. Fool me once, shame on you. Fool me twice, shame on me.

Recently, I'd been trying mightily to protect myself by setting up boundaries, carefully identifying the behaviors I would not be repeating in order to keep myself out of harm's way. Making a baby quilt with Chinese motifs was just asking for trouble, for example. I wasn't taking one step out into Herb's rodent-riddled garden until he plowed it up and smoothed out the paths. I'd be the one with the broken ankle, paying the price. Then I'd vowed never again to set foot on the maple floor of the Linn-Benton Community College gym for Cowboy Dancing.

The trouble here? I was making all these resolutions with a brain prone to dark distortion. My time-honored strategy wasn't working. What seemed obvious one day could look entirely different the next.

I was making a baby quilt after all. The possibility of a broken ankle had not been enough to detour me from gathering ruby red fall raspberries from Herb's treacherously pock-marked garden. And only days after the Great Cowboy Dancing Debacle, going back didn't seem at all like the worst idea in the world.

Finding Dr. Spaulding's office was almost as difficult as securing the appointment in the first place. I'll spare you the details; just know that it seriously made me wonder how anyone ever gets set up for help with drug addiction.

Now I wandered between the dentists' offices, counseling services and physical therapy clinics until I finally stumbled onto it, hiding in plain sight in what had obviously once been a split-level family house.

The receptionist in the desk area that had probably been the kitchen said it was her first day, so my pre-arrangement to pay $200 up front for an hour's consultation seemed to throw her. She handed me a clip-boarded intake form requesting all the usual medical info, plus pages of questions about my addictions and the addictions of my family. I took a seat in the sunken-living room/waiting area.

None, none, none, I scribbled, drawing lines though some of it. Somebody on the phone had already obtained all this info anyway. Couldn't I for once break a few inapplicable rules?

Nothing doing. When I tried to hand it in, she said sorry, I had to complete it fully.

"But a lot of this really just isn't relevant for me." The agreement to be monitored, for example. To accept phone calls reminding me of appointments I wouldn't be making.

"Sorry." She handed it back to me.

Not her fault, but I was hating this. Hating that I had to be here. This house-as-a-medical-office reminded me of one of those weird dreams where death is a motel room. I was shaking. The time for my appointment passed. I was nervous. I had to go to the bathroom. The receptionist pointed me down the hall.

Oh, great. Over the toilet was a sign warning that I was on camera. Well, I had to go. What were my choices?

Back in the waiting room I fidgeted, debating whether to just march up there and ask for my check back and walk out. By the time they called me up, I had to go to the bathroom again.

It took me a minute to realize the woman standing there bare-foot, in cords, a flowered shirt and a fedora, was indeed the long-sought Dr. Spaulding. Maybe her casual attire was disarming for others, but it didn't do anything for me. Apparently I still longed for the white coat which I had previously associated with wisdom.

"I need to use the bathroom before we go in," I said. "But you know, you have a camera in there."

"Yup."

"It's...." I winced. "Kind of demeaning."

"Well, if we didn't do that, people would bring in somebody else's pee for their tests. I'm sorry, but that's my practice."

In the exam room—formerly a bedroom—she listened to my story. I told her I'd taken up to 60 mg of Oxycodone a day for twelve weeks.

She looked up from her clipboard. "Did you ever crush and snort it?"

I shuddered. "No." She had to ask, I suppose. I had a drug prob-lem; I was under suspicion. Never would there be an end to insisting one more time for the record that I had never taken one pill more, one pill sooner than what the doctors ordered.

"The surgeon's taper plan would have had me on it a lot lon-ger," I said, pulling out the chart Herb had made on which I'd plotted my decreasing doses at Christmas the previous year. Fifty milligrams to nothing in three weeks.

"Wow." She studied the chart. Then she grinned. "Nobody does this. Do you mind if I make a copy? I want to show it to my staff."

I appreciated this, somebody recognizing I'd succeeded at something difficult.

"I figured if I took it slower like he said, it would just be that much longer my brain was frying in the stuff."

"You were probably right about that. No, that's good."

Then I told her about the Xanax, and how I'd been off that just two months.

"I think my worst symptom is these horrible mood swings."

"Oh, yeah."

"I mean, I can see I'm taking things much harder than I should, but I don't seem to have any control. And when I spiral down I just feel so desperate. I suppose this is how people are feeling when they relapse."

"Well, exactly."

"Also I'm super tired most of the time. And I get these weird pains down the back of my thighs."

What a relief to have her nod knowingly in recognition at this.

"So these *are* withdrawal symptoms?"

"Oh yeah, for sure."

"Well, when I told my regular doctor about this in August, she said that as far as she knew, anything I still had going on eight months after going off Oxycodone must be something else."

The doctor smiled, shut her eyes, shook her head.

"I guess that's really why I'm here. I thought it would help to have it confirmed that what's going on with me *is* about the drugs. It's enough trying to live through this without worrying I've got some other weird disease coming on."

She nodded. "In general, the opioid withdrawal symptoms tend to be more physical and the benzos are more about the brain."

That sounded right. My nervous anxiety had ratcheted up when I jumped from the Xanax.

I told her about my sinus pain and how I figured it had been so much worse back when it started in March because of hyperalgesia. She nodded, then yanked the exam table's protective paper over the slide-out footrest and clicked open a pen.

"Okay, here's what's going on." She started sketching what looked like little broccoli sprouts. "These are the receptors in your brain. There's one for dopamine, your body's own feel-good neurotransmitter. When all that Oxycodone flooded in, these receptors wake up and you feel really good…"

I shook my head. "Not me. I never got high. Nothing close."

"Well, then you must have just had the whole load going to fight some really massive pain."

Her sketch and explanation were quite complex. I wondered if her other patients were smarter than I, because I wouldn't have wanted to be taking a graded test on this afterwards. I decided that while her get-up may not have registered as professional to me, she really did know her stuff.

"Then when you stop with the drugs," she continued, "your brain's all confused. The receptors have kind of shriveled up and they aren't producing what they're supposed to."

I nodded. I'd read this before. I understood the gist of it.

But then she made it personal and blunt.

"Your brain has been damaged," she said. "You have an iatrogenic disease. That means it was caused by a doctor."

The way she popped up with that—iatrogenic—made me think mine wasn't the first case she'd seen where the word was applicable.

"Your brain will heal, but it takes time."

"But how long? This article on the internet said *two years* from the time of going off the drugs. Tell me that can't be right."

"Well, when did you go off again?"

"New Year's Eve was my last dose of Oxycodone and I quit the Xanax toward the end of August."

"I'd say if you're sleeping okay, you're probably past the worst of the Xanax withdrawal. But for the opioids....you're probably looking at a few more months. The only thing I can't really ascribe to withdrawal would be this sinus headache pain."

"Yeah?" I didn't really want to hear this.

"You might want to consider getting a CAT scan."

I drew back. No way. CAT scans use a lot of radiation. The sinus issue had arisen in conjunction with withdrawal. I figured if all my other withdrawal symptoms went away and I was still stuck with this, *then* maybe I'd pursue it.

Because that's the thing about waiting for your central nervous system to heal—your entire body is affected. So many random sharp pains, for example. You couldn't begin to go chasing down each one down individually. You'd probably give yourself cancer with all the x-rays.

While we'd been swapping furniture around at the beach house I'd had two days of disturbing chest pains. But my heart had always checked out fine in the past. I was chalking it up to withdrawal. And okay, maybe right here is a good place for the disclaimer that obviously I have no business advising anybody else with chest pains to avoid the ER. But this is how I advised myself, and in the end, I was right. The chest pains had gone away.

Now Dr. Spaulding offered acupuncture, but for that I already had Rose Tian with her Chinese music and camera-free bathrooms.

"I'd be happy to set you up with one of our counselors," she said. "We have a great batch of people, and every one of them is a former addict."

I looked down. Noticed again her unencumbered toes. What could I say? I didn't want to sound like I thought I was superior to other addicts, I just didn't see how they could help me. I didn't need anybody to encourage me not to "use" again.

So, a few more months of symptoms she'd said. Herb and I debated this. What exactly did a few mean? I thought at least three, no more than five.

It didn't matter, ultimately. I ended up struggling so far beyond her prediction.

CHAPTER 23

One morning in late October, I was surprised to wake up feeling halfway decent. Since it wasn't raining, I put on my Carhartts and boots, took up my long-handled pruning saw, and headed out to the Doug firs to do a bit of limbing and torch a burn pile.

This trusty saw of mine had turned out to be the best birthday present Herb ever gave me, and I've been through several blades. Technically, tree farmers limb trees to promote clear-grained growth by removing the branches that form knotholes, but I'm never thinking that far ahead. I'm not worrying about producing a superior grade of lumber when the trees are cut down. Maybe they never will be anyway. I just enjoy the immediacy of getting rid of the dead branches and creating vistas through the grove. It feels like artwork to me, framing a picture of the sun hitting a meadow on the far side of the river.

Kind of a silly hobby, Miles called it one time.

Do you think I care about his verdict on this? No, I do not. Engaged in this, I'm happy, content to be alone with my thoughts in the fresh air. It's during my treasured woods time, mind wandering, that I've heard the various characters of my novels talking in my head, demanding to be heard.

Suddenly that day, out in the fir trees, I realized the character in my head who wouldn't shut up was me.

I had to sit down on my rickety lawn chair, astonished.

My brain felt....like it was healing. Like the word itself—*healing*—the the way it rolled off the tongue. Like some thick, rich, calming balm had been smoothed over all those frazzled and freaking-out neurotransmitters.

Suddenly, for the first time, I could clearly see what bad shape I'd been in the past year. I really *had* been put through hell. I'd been feeling absolutely terrible about myself. But—key, here—I was looking *back*.

Words started pouring into my head. I had to tell this story. People should be warned what can happen. They needed to know how fast opioid painkillers could get their hooks in you even if you aren't a person with any sort of predisposition toward addiction.

That night we went to Cowboy Dancing and learned the Sweetheart Shuffle.

For three days I enjoyed the thrill of conception. I had a book in my brain, wanting to grow and be born. I actually jotted a few notes.

And then the window closed.

First the ominous creep of the burning nerve pain in the back of my thighs, the heavy brain fog, the horrifying realization that it would require a huge act of will simply to refrain from bursting into tears.

I lay on the sofa with my heating pad under my thighs. I'd read books saying post acute withdrawal symptoms were signs your brain was recovering. Ha! Seemed to me like the exact opposite, more like reminders that my brain was still limping along, only occasionally coming up with the needed feel-good neurotransmitters.

Also, I was advised that resenting my symptoms would just make me feel worse.

Well, I did resent them. I was angry. Angry at the doctors who let this happen to me. Angry at the current state of addiction medicine and mental health care in our country that offered nowhere to turn.

Wallowing in self-pity is so unattractive. We're taught we must never sink to this. I must confess, lying there completely compromised in mind and body, I did feel sorry for myself. My brain had been hijacked, and however wild a ride the demented pilot devised, I was never allowed the immediate fix of the opioid/benzo oxygen mask dangling in my face. I was entirely alone on this plane and, short of wrenching open the emergency door and flinging myself into the ether, all I could do was hang tight and reach for the barf bag.

One thing seemed clear. I would not be writing a book about all this until I was looking back on it as a person recovered.

At least recovered longer than three days a month.

News stories of our country's epidemic of opioid abuse and addiction now caught my attention at every turn. People addicted to painkillers by prescription were one piece of this big horrible puzzle that was only now becoming clear.

And I was part of it.

Entire West Virginia hamlets of young people who'd never before done more than swig beer becoming swiftly addicted and lost to Oxycodone; celebrities thought to have been clean relapsing and dying of heroin overdoses. Cruel stories of babies born addicted.

Welcome to the world. I couldn't stand the thought of an innocent infant having to endure what I'd been going through.

Alarmed by news stories and patient outcome studies, many doctors went on the defensive. They felt victimized, caught between federal regulators trying to tighten up the flow of narcotics, and the angry, desperate patients insisting the valve, at all costs, be kept open. Doctors no longer "comfortable" continuing the opioid prescriptions they themselves had initiated dismissed patients to newly established pain clinics. Let somebody else try to undo the damage.

A scholarly paper on-line described a study attempting to identify which patients will be likely to abuse painkillers post-surgery. People with prior histories of drug abuse? A higher level of stated *fear* of pain? A higher reported level of *actual* pain? Another article advised, before prescribing, to watch patients for low self-esteem, histories of anxiety or depression. As if the problem of addiction—or at least the physician's responsibility—could be solved simply by identifying ahead of time who's at risk, all the better to flag the patients best avoided from the outset.

Why aren't more researchers studying the mechanism of addiction to opioids itself, the harm these drugs might do to anyone, regardless of their history? Don't people like me who go into surgery without undue trepidation and in possession of sufficient self-esteem still deserve a heads-up?

In areas where access to the meds had been tightened and those addicted by prescription were cut off from their source of supply, emergency rooms had been flooded with people desperate to stop the agony of withdrawal. Journalist Barry Meier details just such a scenario which unfolded in Washington State in his long form piece, *A World of Hurt: Fixing Pain Medicine's Biggest Mistake.*

My own Immediate Care Clinic posts a sign warning of their policy against prescribing narcotics. Don't be telling them you've lost your meds or had them stolen. They know better. Further, they don't deal with tapering plans or the effects of withdrawal.

So, who does, then? Nobody at our clinic, anyway.

Could we have some compassion, please? A little less rush to judgment? These are very sick people. Who knows how innocently they may have taken that first pill?

What interested me most were the posted comments following the on-line articles. It was the people dependent on their prescribed painkillers who wrote the most passionate and panicky rants: *Look how bad things were already. They were having to go to more than one doctor already to get a sufficient supply. This was criminal. Doctors who wouldn't give them their meds were unsympathetic jerks who had no conception of the daily pain they endured, pain they wouldn't wish on their worst enemy.* (A popular phrase.) *Anyone could see the real problem was the true addicts, the filthy junkies, making it so hard for the people with legitimate pain, people like the posters themselves, who had their doctor's prescription to prove their solid moral grounding. Why were they being punished for the pathetic weakness of all these drug abusers?*

People who took their first Oxycodone on a doctor's orders were always deeply defensive at the notion of anyone categorizing them as addicted. As if what was going on in their body in terms of developing tolerance to the meds and increased pain due to hyper-algesia was some process entirely separate from what goes on with *real* addicts. They were not interested in new studies showing that long-term prescribing of opioids for chronic pain is ineffective, that patients, in fact, often end up registering *higher* levels of pain in the long run. Their sole concern was that the doctors not be prevented from keeping their pain meds coming. If they couldn't get the drugs through their doctors, what would distinguish them from all the real addicts, the nasty street junkies? They clung to those prescriptions as if they should serve as a guarantee they would never be asked to face the reality of their own addiction.

That's a mountain of denial to overcome, and I found these stories heartbreaking.

Getting off these drugs would be a huge challenge even if these people could see compassionate help at hand.

Which of course they can't, because it isn't.

Admit you've got a problem with drugs and what do you get? Treatment that feels suspiciously like punishment. No wonder people fight like hell to avoid being stuck with the label of drug addict.

Please. Go ahead.

Show me a suffering person who was ever healed by a sentence of scorn.

Making the baby quilt had ultimately been good for me, especially the soothing process of the final hand stitching in red thread for good luck, Chinese-style. Now the quilt and the Osh Kosh overalls were wrapped and ready for the upcoming baby shower along with Herb's gift, one which would surely eclipse anything anyone else might present. He'd spent many pleasant hours searching out and loading onto the baby's own iPod all the best lullabies, quiet time music, and goofy Raffi songs. He found a song in Chinese which Ziwei would later confirm every Chinese child knows which is called, roughly translated, "Only Mommy is the Best." The Raffi lullaby, "Baby Dear," seemed like an entire family's promise of loving support, and reduced me to tears every time it came on, especially the line about the future "clean and bright." My favorite though, was a catchy number sung by Elizabeth Mitchell—"Who's My Pretty Baby?" I liked picturing myself well enough to someday swoop up that pretty baby of ours and dance him around the house.

I just needed to find one more item—the special mobile we'd hung over Miles's own crib. Maybe presenting it as a gift would help prevent another painful attack of Heirloom Rejection.

So where had I stashed it? I tore the house apart, not bothering to put back what I'd dug out, just hurrying on to the next potential spot. Various closets. The drawer of the antique wardrobe. The cedar chest at the foot of our bed, the one where I kept all the vintage baby clothes. I grew increasingly frantic, and the fact that I was sifting through all the tissue-wrapped homemade clothes Miles had worn but Ziwei didn't want wasn't improving my mood.

I wanted to see us as people who had it together; obviously, we didn't. Our house was a neglected mess. Not dirty—it was just that, living here since the day we were married, we'd never been through the purge required in moving. We had forty years of accumulated stuff and now, look, I couldn't even put my hands on something as important as this mobile!

It was a simple little yellow contraption that revolved smiling wooden bears and honeycombs around a honey pot. With no relevance whatsoever to bears or honey, the tinkling theme song it played was, "It's a Small World After All." We had a faded photo of baby Miles grinning up at it. When we first took him to Disneyland at the age of three, Small World was his favorite ride. I interviewed him on tape at the time, and when I asked him to describe it he said, "The dolls sang and they had costumes....like Chinese!" He never mentioned any other nationality. And then he grew up, and went off to China to find his true love. Small world, indeed!

"Oh my God, Herb, I just remembered. I'm pretty sure I gave it to him already. Yeah, at his birthday. No, no wait. At that last little barbecue they had at the Jackson Avenue house. Jeez, my brain!"

Just one more of all the mental glitches I'd suffered over the past year. Does this make me sound like an unreliable narrator?

I emailed Miles and explained my frantic search: If you tell me you have it, I can at least quit tearing the house apart. I begged for a quick answer, but it was Halloween and he and Ziwei had their hands full, happily handing out candy to hoards of trick-or-treaters in their new, family-friendly neighborhood.

He didn't write back until ten: **Unfortunately, I don't have an answer that'll clear things up; I don't remember you giving us that, and Ziwei doesn't either. I vaguely remember the one you mean.** He promised to look through the boxes in his garage the next day, the ones that hadn't been entirely unpacked during their move, but in the meantime he hoped I wouldn't get so worked up about it.

Well, I *was* worked up. I could see that, watching myself. This was my sick brain making a much bigger deal of something that didn't need to be so painful. But I couldn't help it. Miles's casual attitude made me feel he didn't care about this treasured little token of his childhood that meant so much to me. I could picture him setting it aside with just a brief glance after I'd handed it to him. Maybe he mistakenly put the flat box in with the recycling. Oh, I couldn't *stand* the idea of it going permanently missing after I'd saved it all these years!

In a new sign of an incremental bit of healing on my brain's part, though, when Miles's search failed to turn up the mobile, I didn't fall apart. I didn't cry for an hour. I was just recovered enough to apply a little cognitive therapy, try for one little iota of control over the way I framed this for myself. I was proud to report to Madeline at our next meeting that I realized this: The important thing to me about the mobile wasn't the toy itself; it was the story, the connection in my mind between my baby loving his Small World mobile, the Chinese dancing dolls at Disneyland, and then finding a bride in China. Even if the mobile had accidentally gone to the dump, I still had the story.

A few days later, I woke in the grip of withdrawal. I felt like I had the flu, my body stiff and paralyzed with pain. I didn't want to get out of bed. All I could do was cry. And it was the day of the baby shower.

Shit. I didn't want to see people. I didn't want to go over to my mother's house, where it was being held. I felt too fragile. I feared Miles mocking my quilt. I could just see myself falling apart in front of everybody.

"I don't want to go," I whimpered to Herb. "I can't."

My husband cannot stand the treacly admonition to "make a memory," but that doesn't stop him from making them. It had been a brutal learning curve, but he'd finally started catching on to what worked with me and what didn't.

He undressed, got back into bed, and delivered my favorite fix.

Like any fix, it was temporary, but at least it got me to the baby shower, where Miles was surprisingly sweet about the quilt.

I didn't mind at all the later discovery that Herb had quietly sent Miles a warning heads-up email with the suggestion he be sure to give me kid-glove treatment during the opening of our gifts.

I actually welcomed the evidence of this loving conspiracy to avert a public meltdown on my part.

It seemed like exactly what I'd been needing all along.

CHAPTER 24

Once more I went back to see Dr. Miller. I figured the least I could do for myself was make sure my thyroid wasn't giving me grief again. The symptoms of hypothyroidism are similar to what I was dealing with in opioid withdrawal—lethargy, moodiness, depression. Withdrawal was challenging enough; I couldn't see making myself fight any extra battles.

My planned appeal was derailed when the nurse took my blood pressure: Systolic 160! Good grief. Dr. Miller came in and got busy trying to calm me down, promising nobody was going to diagnose me with hypertension on one reading. I should buy a cuff and calmly start keeping an eye on it.

Calmly? Right.

"I suppose the Propranolol was just keeping it down all these years then?"

"That could be," she said. "Now, you were on Propranolol for anxiety, right?"

"No!" We'd been through this. "It was for preventing migraines." Until Xanax, I'd never had a true anxiety attack in my life, yet look how quickly I could be slapped with this default diagnosis. "So if I have high blood pressure will I have to go back on Propranolol?"

"No, we'd try you on something else."

"Why's that?"

"Well, because of the bad dreams you said it gave you."

"Oh." I sat back, placated by her remembering that part of my story.

I told her about going to Dr. Spaulding and how she'd confirmed my symptoms as classic withdrawal.

"Well, I don't deal with the type of patients Susan has, but I've certainly had plenty of people go off the drugs you've been on without having all these extended neurological symptoms."

The type of patients Susan has. Hear what you will in this. I heard *hardcore junkie types.*

She frowned. "So, does anyone else in your family have this addictive thing going on?"

"But I *don't* have the addictive thing going on. It's not hard for me to not take the stuff. It's just hard for me to feel lousy all the time."

"Okay, well then, does anybody else have this…*sensitivity*?"

I shrugged helplessly. How could we know? Who in my family had ever been put to this test? We'd all gone through our share of surgeries and accidents, but it's only been in the past fifteen years that well-intentioned doctors began the so-called War on Pain, prescribing heavy-duty opioids after things like C-sections and wisdom tooth extractions.

"The only thing Susan said she couldn't associate with opioid withdrawal was this sinus pain thing I've had going on."

Dr. Miller wrapped the blood pressure cuff around my arm again and pumped.

Reading the dial, she gave me a wry smile. "Still right up there."

I left feeling like a ticking time bomb. Of all the things doctors know and don't know, one thing's for sure, right? Walking around with high blood pressure is bad.

I unloaded all this to Madeline that afternoon, fidgeting on her sofa like the nervous wreck I was.

"You know," she said, "listening to your story these past months got me thinking about several of my other patients. I'll have somebody whose mood swings have suddenly gotten way worse and I'll say, 'Didn't you just have surgery recently?' And they'll be like, 'But that was three months ago.' Now I'm wondering if they were going through some opioid withdrawal."

Oh, my God, I loved her for this. For listening to me. For believing me, not just looking for a way to blame me. For caring enough about her other patients to try to put two and two together and figure out something that might actually help.

Isn't this what all doctors ought to be doing?

Too panicky over my blood pressure to wait for another appointment to try a different med, I popped a tab of my remaining Propranolol that night. Better the devil I knew than the one I didn't.

But I'd forgotten how tired Propranolol makes me feel initially. I lay in bed in the middle of the afternoon the next day, completely defeated. I'd liked the way my heart had been beating as it should while off the drug. I felt more alive, less sluggish. Going back on the beta-blocker meant giving up the hope that a speeded-up metabolism might help me lose weight. But, everybody knows high blood pressure leads to strokes and heart attacks. I guess I'd just have to resign myself to being plump.

The Propranolol worked. At the gym I stuck my arm in the cuff and was gratified to see a nice low number.

But something way more interesting happened: my eight-month headache went away.

Go figure. I got out my charts. Yes, I'd been perfectly well aware that the Headache From Hell the previous spring had hit the very day I had finally tapered to nothing on the Propranolol, but since I was taking this drug for migraine prevention, not blood pressure, I'd noticed only that my migraine meds weren't touching it. I had no idea my blood pressure might have been unleashed.

Now I had to wonder about all those times when somebody had hurt my feelings and made my face hurt. Was that just my blood pressure spiking? Maybe the fact that my face *hadn't* hurt the day I first sat there and told my story to Madeline was all about the calming effect of her empathetic listening.

Made as much sense as anything else.

While every horrible downswing seemed as bad as the last when I was in the middle of it, looking back I can see that my crash that night after Cowboy Dancing marked the last of the episodes where I felt I was in the pit purely because a loved one had shoved me there.

Sometimes now I'd have a less than pleasant exchange with Herb or Miles, and afterwards I'd think—*Wait a minute—isn't this where I'd be flipping out?*

And when I did go downhill emotionally, it seemed clearer it was strictly about my brain chemicals.

Herb was catching on too. He felt terrible about our fights the previous summer.

"I just didn't understand that it was about your brain," he said simply.

He found it easier to comfort me when I didn't seem to be blaming every last thing on him. He discovered the effectiveness of *not* trying to argue me out of my despair. A better technique was simply to lie down beside me and wrap me in his arms.

I remember the first time I noticed this. I was sobbing uncontrollably when he got me in a spoon-hold and started stroking my arm. Within a couple of minutes, I shut up. I just stopped crying. Suddenly I didn't feel so bad.

It was probably my brain getting a shot of oxytocin, the bonding hormone.

But go ahead and call it love.

Still, I swear, time in the pit never got any easier. Now my morbid anger wasn't directed so much at my family as it was at the medical system that had set me up, condemned me to go through this. It felt like a prison sentence and for what? I'd followed all their rules.

I cried in memory of all the hospital staff members who reminded us over and over to take our meds on time, and never uttered one warning word about the dangers of addiction. What, were they worried about insulting us? I was mad as hell at the surgeon who'd prescribed the painkillers, mad at his assistant, who'd been justifiably alarmed at the dose and duration of the Oxycodone I was being prescribed, but whose mean, ham-handed manner of doing her job had been a curse on me. I wanted to rewind, rewrite her dialogue. If only she'd been kind. If only her concern about my dosages had been about me, the patient, and not the clinic, and whether they'd be running afoul of the law if too many prescriptions for narcotics were linked to them. If only she'd said, *Look honey, I know it hurts, but maybe the pain you're feeling now is partly withdrawal. Let me explain this.....* Never in anything that woman said to me did I hear the slightest hint of sympathy. If only either she or the doctor or somebody at the hospital had given us the actual information we needed, the knowledge that when you taper off Oxycodone, you will feel pain. We should have been warned that waiting for the pain to stop before quitting the pills can only lead to addiction.

If only, if only....what about the whole concept of informed consent? I had not been properly informed!

"It doesn't do any good," Herb would say, "to lie there and cry and be mad at the doctors all over again."

Like I was crying as a thought-out strategy toward good health? I was crying because I felt horrible. And please, I'd heard the drill about forgiveness. Everybody knows you can't heal emotionally if you don't forgive the people who've hurt you. In the middle of the horrors of withdrawal, though, to be condescendingly invited to remember you've been victimized by cluelessness and not pure vindictive evil is no comfort at all. At the bottom of the pit, forget forgiveness—I was mad.

"You're just making it worse," Herb kept insisting.

Oh, yeah, worse for him, sure. But maybe I had to cry. If I didn't, I'd explode. Maybe this was the kind of anger that makes a man grab a gun and go out and see if he can get a cop to help him commit suicide. Women? We just lie there in that dark place and struggle against ourselves. I felt like I was periodically orchestrating my own psych ward, trying to keep safe from myself while also staying clear of the folks up at the hospital who might shoot me full of calm-down drugs first and ask questions later. I never needed anyone actually physically restraining me from killing myself. I needed the people who loved me to hear my distress and tell me why I mattered to them. Give me some warming words to hang onto when I was down in the black pit.

After going through this so many times, I eventually came to wonder if this is why people make the attempts that don't actually finish themselves off, but do get them hauled to the hospital. Maybe, like me, they don't really want to be dead, but can't think how else to let people know the degree of desperation they're feeling. As for those who succeed, stories of suicides now distressed me as never before. Still do. I cannot bear the judgmental commentaries offered up by others about the selfishness or cowardliness of those who take their own lives. I can think only of those poor souls trapped in such a horrifying darkness that killing themselves could seem like a reasonable escape.

I resented Herb adding his voice to the keening chorus I imagined, everybody tut-tutting, lamenting the way I was handling this so poorly. I would lie there sobbing, fantasizing. I wanted to hear him on the phone giving the doctor hell. *I want my wife back, you SOB! She used to be so happy and productive and got so much done around here I called her a Total Force of Nature, and now, thanks to you, she's a sniveling wreck!*

Wasn't going to happen. Would *never* happen. And this feeling that I'd been left to forever act as my own advocate when I was too weak and beaten down to take on the role would be my PTSD trigger for a long time to come.

"Can you pick up some more of that Apple Crunch bread?" I'd beg Herb from the sofa, giving in to my only true craving. It seemed to help, but was I just stupidly making myself fat, eating cake/bread, when simply going back on Lexapro—the Selective Serotonin Reuptake Inhibitor—might give me the same relief, the same increase in serotonin, but in a steady, calorie-free way?

My goal, though, was a clean brain, not to mention having developed a particular antipathy for this drug I suspected of being the reason I had to take so much Oxycodone in the first place. Also, anecdotal evidence indicated that just because I'd had no trouble going off it before didn't mean it would necessarily work so easily for me again. And some people did experience a lot of withdrawal symptoms. Why flirt with that? Besides, this wasn't regular depression, these intermittent attacks of despair. In between them I sometimes felt fine. And now that I'd had a few windows of true mental clarity and health, I hated the idea of losing that by reaching for the leveling agent.

I had to cling to those windows, those brief times when the clouds would part and a ray of light would shoot through. On those days, it was as if I were being visited by this person from the past: Me.

I liked her. She was confident. Energetic. She had better things to do than lie around crying. I wished she'd come around more often. I wanted her back for good.

CHAPTER 25

On December 3rd, 2013, I received an email from the Beckham Center for Orthopedics & Sports Medicine:

Like them on Facebook to Enter for a Chance to Win a Kindle Fire HD!

CHAPTER 26

———————◆

I called my old college roommate in Nebraska and asked if, in her practice as a social worker, she'd ever dealt with anyone going through opioid withdrawal.

Of course she hadn't. I was getting the picture: people trying to recover from opioid addiction tended to land with more specialized rehab counselors.

I told her what I'd been going through and shared the good news of our impending grandparenthood.

"But, Cathy, I need to get well! I want to be part of the solution here, not part of the problem."

"Well then," she said in the wonderfully calm way she had, "you're just going to be that."

Sounded so wise, but I wasn't off the phone five minutes before I remembered: withdrawal just doesn't work that way. I couldn't just ignore these sudden assignments to go directly to the DIY psych ward, nor could I schedule them around whatever else was on the calendar.

I was not in control. The drugs and the damage they'd left behind still were.

I expressed the same concern about being well in time for the baby to my friend Tess, and she wrote back with a warmly supportive letter that ended like this: **I look at that great picture of you by your burn pile on that rare good day and I just have to believe that's the real you, and that bit by bit, you WILL win this awful battle. And maybe even sooner than you think, with that precious baby just a few weeks from being in your arms!! I know how much you want to feel one hundred percent well by then, but even if you're not quite there yet when the big day comes, that little guy is going to bring so much joy to every atom of you—every muscle and bone and fiery little synapse, every blood cell pumping through that great heart of yours—that all of that (plus the right dose of your thyroid medicine!)—will smash every ache and pain and bad feeling and have the bad days on the run before you know it, that's what.**

I cried to read this. I so wanted her beautiful and encouraging words to be true. But I was afraid I'd fail. Even the miracle of birth might not overcome the sad, sick depletion of all the feel-good neurotransmitters in my brain if the great event came on a day that found me down in the pit. What a loser, if even life's greatest miracle couldn't heal me.

Okay, wait. I had to re-frame this:

A baby was coming.

I would get well.

Neither of these things would be any less wonderful for not arriving simultaneously. Time to take a deep breath, keep living this story, see for myself how it would all turn out.

On the tenth day back on Propranolol, I had the first snake dream. On the eleventh, the second. On the twelfth, jerking awake three times in the night, I took it as proof positive.

How many spiders had dropped from the ceiling over the years? How many snakes had slithered under our covers? *Quick quick gotta get away from it...I know I do this but this is different.... this time it's real......* How many panicky hallucinations had freaked us awake?

Linda's silly, quirky brain; that had always been the story.

But now I knew: there was nothing wrong with my brain at all.

It was the damned drug.

And I wasn't going to take one more dose.

As soon as I stopped it, the sinus headache came right back. Bingo. Another hypothesis proved. Blood pressure spikes had been giving me headaches. Too bad I had to figure this out for myself. Too bad it took me so long.

I woke up in pain and, from the bed, asked Herb to call Dr. Miller's at eight on the dot. Maybe we could manage to snag one of the slots we'd figured out they keep open for people needing to come in that day.

Yes. We got one.

Herb drove us to Philomath over the snow-packed highway. Dr. Miller prescribed Verapamil, a different blood pressure medication. Wanting to start it right away, I was disappointed our pharmacy had none in stock, and I'd have to wait.

"I have to tell you something," Herb said that afternoon, back home. "But I don't want you to get upset."

Oh, right. As if the uttering of those words ever did anything but shoot fear straight to my heart.

"I think I may need to go back to the doctor's. I've been having this pain and it's getting worse. It feels like the kidney stone thing."

Oh, no. Herb had suffered three or four similar attacks in the past, but had been fine since a corrective surgery some fifteen years earlier. Strictly rearview-mirror business, we'd thought.

"I'm going with you," I said when he reported he'd managed a late afternoon appointment.

"You don't have to."

"Yes, I do."

With Herb driving the truck and me the Subaru, we caravanned our way over the ice to Miles's and Ziwei's. Regretfully, we had to cancel coming to the goose dinner Miles was planning for us that night. (Yes, our son can cook a goose Chinese-style!) Instead, we left them the Subaru. It had started snowing around December 6th, and our snow-plowless town was still paralyzed. Miles didn't have a four-wheel drive vehicle, and Ziwei's doctor had been saying she might go into labor at any time.

"Do you want me to drive?" I asked Herb. The sun was angling beautifully over the sparkly white world, a novelty in our land of rainy gray winters. "You know I can drive the truck."

"No. It keeps my mind off the pain." He wanted to stop and buy the heating pad he knew from experience he was going to need to tough this out.

"Honey, you can use mine. My legs aren't even hurting today." I'd been dragging the heating pad around for months, trying to soothe whichever part of me needed it. But today—maybe it was the adrenalin—I wasn't in any pain.

"No, I'm not going to take yours," he said, steering over the ice into the Safeway parking lot.

That wasn't the point anyway, I knew. He wanted control. He wanted to buy something that might help.

I couldn't stand watching him stumping around the store in pain, insisting on checking for himself in each aisle. I ran ahead, doing the female thing—asking—quickly ascertaining that Safeway did not carry what we wanted. Next door at BiMart I did the same, speeding up the process, and soon we were on our way toward the doctor's in Philomath again, heating pad in hand.

"See this?" Herb tapped a knob on the dashboard. "This puts it into four-wheel drive. Turn it this way to take it out."

"Couldn't I just leave it in?"

"No, you'll wreck the truck if you use it when you shouldn't."

Without saying, I knew we were discussing the possibility of me ending up driving him across town and up the hill to the hospital. We'd been through this before with his earlier kidney stone episodes. The treacherous roads now, though, put a whole new spin on it. Perhaps literally.

The doctor quickly, sympathetically diagnosed Herb as having a classic presentation of a kidney stone. He'd had this himself and knew just how bad it felt.

Herb paced as we waited alone in the room for the results of the urinalysis.

"So, do *you* think this has anything to do with stress?" I said. The doctor had flatly said no, but Herb's three earlier episodes had every last one occurred when I was out of town speaking at teachers' conventions. He'd never seemed the slightest bit uneasy about holding the fort with the three kids on his own, but neither of us had ever been able to dismiss the coincidence either.

"I found some stuff on the internet this afternoon," he said. "A study that *did* link stress to kidney stones. All I know is, when I felt that pain, the first thought that crossed my mind was *No, this can't happen now. I have to take care of everybody.*"

Poor Herb. He really had been trying to function full-time as the sole family rock.

We waited. The clinic seemed quiet; everyone else had gone home. How many times in the course of our marriage had we sat together in some doctor's exam room waiting, one or the other of us hurting?

My mind raced with scenarios. If Ziwei went into labor, maybe I'd have to show up at the hospital without Herb. But how could I do that? I wouldn't want to leave him alone....

Finally the doctor returned with results confirming his diagnosis. He handed Herb a prescription:

Oxycodone.

The next afternoon I sat in Madeline's office dramatizing all this for her. We'd ended up counting it as something of a Christmas miracle, the speed with which Herb was able to pass that bit of "gravel" and recover. Our kids no longer found amusement in the notion of parents on drugs, and sounded relieved to hear their father had only needed three tabs of Oxy. Herb was fine today, even driving me down to my appointment with Madeline over the icy roads, dropping me off to pick my slow and treacherous way along the slippery sidewalks. I was so glad Ziwei hadn't gone into labor with Miles having to navigate the roads like this, even with our Subaru.

What really struck me about the whole episode, though, was how it had made me feel. For the first time in forever it wasn't *me* who was the sick one, in pain, weak and dependent. Everybody knows how exhausting it can be to take on the role of caregiver, but at least it allows you to retain the self-respect you entirely forfeit as the needy one. Much better to be strong enough to be able to go around taking care of others. Not that I'd had to do anything in the end. Still, the flood of adrenalin that came with knowing I might need to step up had felt so good.

Now that adrenalin had drained away. My legs ached. I was back in the clutches of withdrawal, plus, with my blood pressure uncontrolled again, my sinus was throbbing unmercifully. The pharmacy had finally rounded up my new prescription, so when Herb picked me up at an icy curb after my session with Madeline, he had the pills with him. I went home, took the first dose and lay down on the sofa.

Kick in. C'mon, kick in.

I fell into a toxic-nap nightmare, wherein I awoke lying on a gurney that was being wheeled through a dark fog drifting among the trunks of the poplars out in our field. As the light came up, I saw the leaves drifting down golden around me. A frightening shadow figure was pulling the gurney forward. I sat up, panicked. *Who's there? Who is that? Where are you taking me?*

I opened my eyes to the comfort of the flickering Christmas tree lights, Herb's quiet baby-time collection of classical music filling the room.

CHAPTER 27

We awoke the next morning to a message on the phone. Apparently we'd slept through earlier calls. It was Mary:

"Um, Miles tried to call, but you didn't answer. Ziwei's water broke and they're going up to the hospital."

Yikes! We scrambled, Herb more effectively than I. While he phoned Miles, I stood there trying to wrap a gift for my friend Gwen. We'd planned to take her and her husband out for her birthday celebration dinner that night. I like to think it didn't take *too* long before it hit me that, whatever happened about the baby, we would *not* be going out to dinner that night!

"You'll like this," Herb said. "Miles seems mainly concerned that I come over and finish up his goose soup."

I laughed. Honestly, you can never make up the sort of details real life provides.

"I should go, too," I said. Although I was scared. Maybe I'd watched too many episodes of *Call the Midwife.* Also, I'd heard about the horror of intrusive mothers-in-law. I wasn't sure *what* my role here was supposed to be. This was women's business, right? But it was something I knew nothing about. Three kids, two c-sections; one scheduled due to toxemia, one planned for the twins and initiated when my water broke. I'd never been in labor and was entirely unfit to cheer a person on, even if she'd wanted her mother-in-law there, which I had long ago come to the conclusion she did not.

I walked in expecting to find Ziwei writhing on the sofa. Instead, she was upstairs, showering. She came down combing out her long black hair. Just before they left, she calmly went through her wallet.

"We're supposed to take some cash," she observed, and I grinned at Herb.

Back at our house, I burned some nervous energy by wiring the evergreen garlands I was determined to have up in time for Christmas. I emailed Tess. She'd want to be calling out the angels. I'm always glad to hear my friends are praying on our behalf. Surely they all have more direct connections to God than I.

Before long, I crashed. A wave of withdrawal symptoms hit me, along with the massive migraine I usually get with a rush of relief. The timing of all this had been hanging over us, and the fact that Herb's recovery and the roads thawing into navigable slush had neatly preceded Ziwei's labor had completely done me in.

I lay on the sofa, spiraling downward. Herb put on the baby quiet-time track and gave me the reports as they came. Labor would be goosed along with Pitocin. Later, through the afternoon, Ziwei was having a lot of trouble, a lot of pain.

Oh, God. I fixed my eyes on the twinkling lights twined around the antique angel doll I had on the top of the wardrobe style TV cabinet. *Calling all angels.* Wasn't there some song at the gym with those lyrics? Yes, send in the angels. Ziwei and I needed them. *Help us, save us, deliver us from evil, deliver us from pain.*

I was crying. This was exactly how I *didn't* want this to go. How I'd dreaded it would go. Damn those doctors! They did this to me. I was better off with my arthritic old knee than a new knee and a ruined brain. Almost a whole year since I'd taken a crumb of Oxycodone and here I was, still sick, still weak, still one of the needy ones just when my family needed me to be strong. We didn't need two women in trouble at once.

Around four my migraine meds seemed to kick in. Suddenly, I realized I didn't feel so bad otherwise, either. My legs weren't aching. That's how the withdrawal symptoms worked. They could ambush me one minute, give me a break the next.

As it turned out, Ziwei was doing better too, having been given an epidural right at that time. I'm not reaching for mystical here. Just reporting the facts: when she stopped hurting, so did I.

Miles said they still had a long way to go and there was no use in our coming up to the hospital. He wanted us to go over to their house and check on their cat.

Around eight, though, I told Herb I thought we should go up to the hospital. I wanted to show the family flag while it seemed I could. I couldn't bear the thought of Ziwei having even the briefest thought we were just going about our business, not pulling for her emotionally every step of the way. We phoned to check with Miles.

"Sure, you can come if you want, but Ziwei says she feels bad for you to have to drive all the way across town."

Oh, my God. We're talking five miles. Did she have the slightest clue what this whole thing meant to us? Maybe not. Maybe she wouldn't understand until some distant day when this baby trying to be born was holding vigil at his own laboring wife's side.

Wearing our purple, honored-visitor wristbands, we found our way through the Christmas-decorated halls and crept into the windowless womb of their hospital birthing room.

All is calm, all is bright.

We'd thought to come bringing reassurance, but the visit did *us* more good than them. They were in capable hands. The epidural was doing such a good job of easing Ziwei's pain, it took me awhile to realize she was having contractions. What, had I thought she'd stopped? Like I said, for a woman with children, I understand very little about labor and delivery.

"Go home and get some sleep," Miles said, and promised to call with the news at whatever hour.

"Seriously," I said. "No matter what time it is. Because I'm often awake at three, and if you haven't phoned because you're thinking you'll let us sleep, I'll just be worrying and wondering what's going on."

Out in the hall, we met the nurse now coming on shift, a pretty young woman with shiny blond hair. I begged her to take good care of Ziwei, explaining that her mother was in China and how I was sure this is all pretty scary for her.

Awake at three, as I'd predicted, with no call, I did the math. Didn't they say one centimeter per hour? And she was at eight when we were at the hospital at nine o'clock. What on earth was going on? I woke Herb and had him text Miles.

Good job, honey, learning to message just in time for this great event, because we were then treated to a texted blow-by-blow account, twenty minutes apart, over the next hours:

They've rolled in a cart of equipment. Looks promising.

Doc's here.

She's pushing.

They feel his head.

Still pushing. Almost there.

And finally, about six in the morning:

He's out!

Minutes later, Miles phoned, relieved and jubilant. In the background I could hear that darling daughter of ours laughing. They were putting the baby to her breast.

"Look at him go for it," I heard the nurse saying.

Oh, nicely staged, this New Age Birth by Text, this immediate phone connection to the purest joy.

Herb and I hugged. I loved our life. I loved our ongoing stories.

A few hours later we walked into the hospital. We knew the way to the maternity ward now. We were old hands. We were grandparents! We passed each nurses station, grinning at everyone, conscious of the glow we must be giving off. Maybe they saw this all the time, but it was brand new for us.

I hope this won't sound like sacrilege. We weren't expecting a Second Coming with the birth of our grandchild. But when we ventured into the shelter of their room, I felt like we were stealing into the manger on bended knee to behold the Holy Family.

Look at the three of them. I especially couldn't get over our son, our baby. What a miracle, the way he'd morphed from a sullen teenager into this tenderly smiling daddy.

Soon enough I found a seat and they laid that little baby boy in my arms.

Oh, my God. Tess was right. Everybody'd tried to warn me and I thought I was prepared, but still it hit me fresh. Look at his little face! Suddenly I knew I wanted nothing else in life going forward but to spend as much time as I could bonding with this baby. Call it oxytocin, call it joy—all those good feelings were indeed coursing through every cell of my body.

Still high, Ziwei was nonetheless stunned at the difficult reality of childbirth, at least as it had played out for her.

"But the nurses were so nice to me," she kept exclaiming, as if surprised she merited any courtesy at all. "This one, she kept saying, 'You are strong! You can *do* this.' And then she kisses me on the forehead."

I was so glad, because for this daughter from China, I felt *responsible* for our medical care system. I was so grateful our prayers had been answered, and an angel of kindness had indeed appeared.

Herb and I fairly flew out of the hospital. We just kept looking at each other. *Are you as astonished as I am?* We hadn't been over-whelmed by so much happiness in years.

For so long now it had seemed like no matter what I did, no matter how hard I tried, the universe was flat-out against me. Now I felt nothing but benevolent approval beaming down from above. Maybe I wasn't such a loser after all. I had convinced a strong and steadfast man to marry me. The two of us had supported each other through all the usual trials, the challenges of children, the decline and death of parents, plus the troubles life had thrown specifically our way—infertility, the time the tree fell on Herb, smashing his spleen, his scary kidney issues, the ever ongoing fallout of my long-ago sewing needle accident. We'd encouraged Miles in this across-the-world courtship, loved Ziwei for loving our son before we ever met her. Now they'd given us this little six-pound miracle. Our family was continuing. And because through it all we'd hung tight, we had arrived at this place together, to share this day of all days.

Only now did I truly understand the significance of the line from Psalm 128 quoted in the souvenir program for my great-grand-parents' fiftieth wedding anniversary:

The Lord shall bless thee—Yea, thou shalt see thy children's children.

"Let's stop downtown," I said. "Let's have lunch out."

We saw no one we knew at New Morning Bakery, but that didn't stop me from bubbling over with our good news to anyone who cared to hear about it. And people did. A baby's always good news for everyone. For the first time in so long I felt joyful and triumphant. Go ahead! Ask me how I'm doing! I finally had something wonderful to report.

That night we resurrected the dinner plans with our friends Gwen and her husband, David, and toasted life itself in celebration.

CHAPTER 28

Unfortunately, my damaged neurotransmitters were not impressed by Life's Oldest Miracle.

Or maybe they were. Maybe they were saying *Hey c'mon—we pumped out the good stuff you wanted for the big day. Now we're shot! Give us a rest already!*

I was back to weeping in the bathtub.

"You *are* getting well," Herb insisted.

"No, I'm not."

"You *are*."

"How can you keep saying that? Every time this happens I feel just as bad as every time before, and it's just *one more time it's happened again*."

He pulled me out, wrapped me in a towel, took me into the bedroom and folded himself around me on the bed.

"I'm *never* going to get well," I wailed. "I'm getting nothing but older and fatter and I'll be completely old and ready to die before I'm ever well. We don't have enough *time!*"

"Shh," he said, stroking my shoulder. "We have all the time we need."

After Christmas, I made what I thought would be my last visit to Madeline. I told her about the baby's birth and how Herb and I had pulled off hosting Christmas for the extended family, even though it meant I'd been interspersing stints of garland hanging with episodes of crashing on the couch. I'm sure I looked perfectly fine to my brother and his family. I was the only one so painfully conscious of myself as a sick person, still subject to these crippling attacks of pain and psychic despair.

I told Madeline Herb's lovely words: *We have all the time we need.*

He doesn't even remember saying them now. I love how every once in awhile he accidentally gets it just right. If he'd said *We have all the time in the world,* I wouldn't have bought it. I'd have argued, outraged. Because we're old enough now that we don't, as they say, have our whole lives in front of us.

I would hang on to the way he'd put it: *All the time we need.*

Have I mentioned how much I love my husband?

I could have kept seeing Madeline forever, but by now my mind had healed enough that I could laugh to think I'd ever thought my marriage was imperiled by the fact that my sweet and loyal husband couldn't help popping his jaw. And that's what had brought me to her office in the first place—my relationships. She really couldn't help me that much with ongoing withdrawal symptoms.

When I got up to leave for a final time, she reminded me I could call her again, and if I needed to, I shouldn't think of it as some kind of defeat.

"You have a beautiful mind," she said, holding the door open for me.

What a nice thing to say. What a lovely parting benediction.

I hope she meant it.

I hope it's true.

So, how much more time *would* we need?

Are you ready for it?

(Thank God for not being able to see into the future.)

Another two years.

New Years 2014 marked twelve months since my last crumb of Oxycodone. I felt no pride at the length of time I'd been "clean." I hadn't been fighting cravings. I couldn't claim amazing willpower. I did not feel a celebration was in order. All I felt was appalled.

I looked back at all the false starts, all the times I'd been dragged down into the pit after having strung together three good days in a row and tentatively calling it the start of being well. Anticipating the baby's birth and worrying about hosting Christmas had completely stressed me out.

I got it now. It didn't matter how busy and productive of a person I used to be. For now, I wasn't that person. I was somebody who needed to have absolutely *nothing* on my calendar.

My diagnosis? Terminally Tentative.

My prescription? The No Plans Plan.

No more setting myself up for feelings of failure, filling a calendar with commitments I'd be unlikely to keep. I was taking a belated Sick Leave. My To-Do list would be put on indefinite hiatus. On good days I'd try to accomplish whatever I could. When the black wave hit, I'd hunker down on the couch with my heating pad and take my frazzled brain to *Downton Abbey.* My mother had given me the series set for Christmas. I would start over at the beginning. Surely I'd be well by the time I finished.

Right. What optimism. Before I was well, I would have to up my Netflix take from three to six disks at a time and watch all nine seasons of *How I Met Your Mother* and the ten years of *Friends,* many episodes watched back-to-back in the middle of fearfully long, dark nights. I caught up on all my favorite TV series plus every old movie I remembered liking as a child.

I canceled a March speaking engagement I'd made almost a year previously for the Convention of the Oregon Council of Teachers of English. No more of this business of thinking *Surely, surely I'll be well by then,* only to be disappointed.

And I told Herb I realized I really didn't care about having a 40th anniversary party in June. Who were we kidding? We're not party people. And we agreed on this: celebrating coming through the worst year of our marriage still together didn't need to be a display any more than getting married forty years ago had been about insisting on some over-the-top, Most-Important-Day-of-Our-Lives Wedding Extravaganza.

One day while I was lying on the sofa taking the *Downton Abbey* cure, Herb came into the living room with a shoebox. He'd been putting the Christmas decorations away.

I paused the show. "What."

He opened the box and pulled it out—the missing Small World mobile.

"Found it in the back of the closet at the top of the stairs."

"Oh, my gosh." I was weepy with delight and, at the same time, bewildered. "This isn't even the box I was picturing it in. Herb, my *brain*. I saw that scene in my head, the business of giving it to Miles, him just setting it aside...and it never happened!"

The funny part was telling Miles. He couldn't believe my delight in being wrong. Wasn't I alarmed about the state of my mind? Actually, as a mother, I preferred knowing my own memory (which would presumably improve) had been the culprit rather than that my son had been as coldly callous as I'd been fearing. And of course I was just so glad this little treasure hadn't accidentally ended up at the dump.

We fastened the mobile to the wooden back of the Stickley couch where it dangled over the bassinet in use here for the sole attendee and star pupil of Wake Robin Farm Daycare and Academy for Exceptional Grandchildren.

He liked it.

Obsessive observer of my own thoughts, I noted the fits and starts of my brain's healing. One day, buying frames for baby pictures, I found myself wandering the craft store aisles, thinking how such places always make me want to do projects. So what should I make? What would be fun to try?

Hey, wait a minute. Where did that come from, such a sparkly little thought? That was my *old* way of thinking.

I wandered over to a bin of To-Do-list pads on sale and fished one up. In the highly decorated Mary Englebrett lettering, I found, just for me, this message: **At any given moment, you have the power to say, "This is not the way the story is going to end."**

I dreamed I was down in the woods in deep snow, struggling to manage a fire of fir boughs. Herb called my cell and I heard his loving voice: *I'm coming to get you out of there right now. I love you and I'm never going to leave you.*

So what if Herb never actually talked this way? Something positive was obviously going on in my brain if it could put out enough of those good chemicals to allow me to imagine it.

My daughter says I have the most transparent dreams she's ever heard recounted. They would be far too obvious in fiction. I had begun the writing of this book, desperate to feel some good could be salvaged from my experience, when I dreamed I had been trudging a long ways around the farm's trees through deep, boot-sucking mud. I climbed the front porch steps and took a seat on the bench. Resting one boot across my other knee, I began picking from the muddy waffle soles one shiny new penny after another. The best part? In spite of the mud, those copper coins were coming out completely clean.

We were Cowboy Dancing drop-outs, thanks to me. We signed up for winter term and agreed we'd go when I felt well, sit it out the other times, no problem. But it *was* a problem. We made fewer than half the classes, and Herb admitted he didn't appreciate feeling he was forever getting behind in learning the new steps. We agreed to skip spring term if he would promise to sign up again in the fall without me having to talk him into it all over again. In the end, it didn't matter; even by then I couldn't commit to a class. Not even the October after that.

I still had seasons to go, hundreds more loops of the trees to do—tiny white daisies at my feet, pink wildflowers, drifting puffs of cottony poplar seeds, grass gone gold by summer, strewn with brown oak and maple leaves by fall, boggy in the winter with the recently risen river and slushy with melting snow.

"I'm ordering this CD about anger and forgiveness," I told Herb. "That make you happy?"

His campaign to argue me out of my simmering anger was definitely in need of some back-up.

While I started listening with a certain defiant resistance—I had every right to be mad!—I was surprised at how comforting this meditation by Belleruth Naparstek turned out to be. How could somebody who hadn't heard my story know so precisely what I would find persuasive? Perhaps it's the acknowledgment that people who've gone through *any* kind of trauma are bound to be saddled with a lot of resentment. I marveled at the cunning elegance in the writing of this script, how gently I was led into the understanding that releasing my rage was definitely going to be for my own benefit.

I see myself jumping on my mini-trampoline in the backyard that summer, calling forth the power of the triple Rx—cardio exercise, the healing magic of the morning sun, and Naparstek's calming voice, backed by an uplifting orchestral soundtrack. Above me, the spreading branches of our sheltering oak.

Off to the right, the garden with the antique screen-door gate, the one with the metal **PIONEER** off some old woodstove or hunk of farm machinery nailed on it. What a thrill, the moment I forked that up out of an overgrown old trash pile out in the woods. It had always meant covered wagons to me, but now, look—I was a pioneer in recovering from iatrogenic addiction. Of course I could be forgiving of the misguided people who'd put me here. Obviously, being well again would feel so good, I'd have no room in my heart for bitterness. No time.

To my left, a lovely, oxytocin-inducing scene: Herb on the patio with the baby, feeding him mashed-up plums from our own trees. I was the floorshow: Grandma Getting Well. And lucky me— what a glorious set-up for rehab, my own beautiful home and land, staffed full-time by the best husband, featuring daily healing visits by Nolan Yin-Nuo (Solemn Promise) Crew, the most charming grand-child ever. I loved seeing this baby's daddy every day too. Herb and I agreed—seeing his enchantment with his little boy was as satisfying as playing with the baby himself.

But I remember, too, afternoons lying on the chaise, staring up into the branches of that same oak, completely shot down, dragged back to the pit. I knew it was all about the *lack* of dopamine or sero-tonin or GABA or whatever in my brain, but it felt like some demon scientist had jabbed a big syringe straight through my skull and deep into my brain, pushing the plunger to release some evil black poi-son. I looked like a woman sprawled on a chaise, but I felt like a lab rat cuffed to a table. *Let's just see if she can be brave enough to stand THIS*.......

No matter how many times I enjoyed periods of feeling perfectly well, I could never seem to escape these brutal attacks of desperation.

Most people have experienced physical pain—a broken bone, a toothache, childbirth. They've endured the flu, or a nasty hangover. So, to the extent you can describe your physical withdrawal symp-toms as something they relate to, fine.

But I still struggle to adequately express in words the grim mental state that can be the result of drug withdrawal. Over and over I could barely understand it myself just a day beyond any given incident. We are talking about taking the mind of a person who has previously fully embraced life, and suddenly downloading into that brain thoughts of making a swift exit. I kept telling Herb that my brain just *hurt*. But, you see? That says nothing; that does not describe it anymore than does the technical term, "chemical depression."

I can report only the appalling thoughts produced by this compromised brain. From the bottom of the black pit, I could not summon an ounce of forgiveness for anyone who'd had the slightest thing to do with putting me there. I remembered everyone I'd confided in along the way, everyone who was apparently not giving a second thought to how my story had turned out. I cursed them.

Did these doctors have the slightest clue the sentence they'd handed me? Here—live through this, all the long months, depressingly sick in mind and body. We'll throw in the occasional good day, allowing you to climb a rung or two of the ladder, but when you slide down yet another chute, your damaged brain will never be able to remember the feeling of those better days, or imagine the possibility of any more of them in the future. Instead, with horrifying relentlessness, you'll keep hearing your own mind's morbid suggestion:

You're a ridiculously sick person and you're never going to get well. Ever. Why don't you just give up and kill yourself?

Only don't.

Try to stay alive.

How hard can that be?

Hard, as it turns out. Appallingly hard.

At my bitterest, I thought, quite simply, I was doing everybody a huge favor by not killing myself. Hadn't I tried to explain the horror of this kind of mental distress? Weren't people who felt this bad supposed to be helped and encouraged?

And I'm not just talking about doctors. I wished that whatever it was my friends and family would kick themselves for not doing if I were to give up, they would do now, when I needed it. Now, when it might help me hang on.

No need to point out these are not nice thoughts. I'm aware of that. And be assured I didn't appreciate having them. But I'm trying to write the truth here, and I need my words to be a testimony to what can happen to a person's mind thanks to the damage caused by physician-prescribed drugs.

I'm grateful to myself for my own stubbornness in clinging to this crucial fact: I did not want to be dead.

CHAPTER 29

On May 20th, 2014, I received another email from the Beckham Center for Orthopedics & Sports Medicine:

Like them on Facebook to Enter for a Chance to Win a Kindle Fire HD!

CHAPTER 30

A four-story luxury apartment building was being built on the Corvallis riverfront, an entirely new concept in a college town where "apartment" and "student housing" were used interchangeably. This would be different. This would be deliberate, sophisticated apartment living for grownups, and I wondered aloud to Herb if it might actually be perfect for my mother.

"Oh, jeez, don't bring it up," Herb said. "You'll just get her upset."

Not an unfair concern. Any hinting of the advantages of moving out of her home of nearly fifty years usually did have that effect.

"But the other day she was saying what she liked about her house is that she can still look out the kitchen window and see the kids walking to school. She's not trying to claim she's not old anymore. She just doesn't want to see *only* old people. At these apartments she could look down and see the whole world going by. They set up the farmer's market right below."

"I still think you're asking for trouble."

Okay, but since when could I ever keep my mouth shut when I thought I had a good idea? Driving my mom up to the Kings Valley cabin for a Mother's Day brunch gathering, I asked her offhand if she'd ever considered being one of the first to move into what they were calling the Jax118.

She did not get upset. Instead, a short three days later, she said, "I've thought about it, and I want to move into those apartments."

Well! I'm a huge fan of decisiveness; I was thrilled. Also, my brain appreciated the good hit of registering that my real estate advice was being valued. True, Mary and Jaci had forwarded a few house-for-sale links during their recent Portland house hunt preceding their move from Corvallis, but I'd been quite conscious of their preference for me to remain in Mouth-Shut Mode.

No surprise, then, that I warmed to this, and I went into high gear, promising my mother she had nothing to worry about. Herb and I knew how to sell houses. We would enlist once again the charming Clare Staton whose mother, in another small town connection, was actually friends with *my* mother. The apartments would be ready for occupancy on Sept 1st, so we'd have the summer to sort and pack Mom's house. I tried to sound as confident as I could while still being painfully aware that my energy levels were, to put it mildly, still wildly variable.

My mother was excited. She told me over and over how much she appreciated me figuring everything out. This was going to be a great new chapter in her life.

I could practically feel the dopamine firing off in my brain. This was the sort of project where I could be "in the flow"—defined as feeling that the task at hand is perfectly suited to one's skill set.

How long had it been since I'd felt remotely competent about anything? I welcomed the rush.

One day while driving my mom down to put her deposit on the apartment, I explained the system of dispersing possessions Herb's family had used with great success. I would take pictures of any item she wanted to part with and send these around to all her grandkids, who would in turn let my brother and me know which item interested them. Then Bob and I would flip a coin for first choice and start dibsing back and forth.

I'd started getting nervous when Mom had seemed inclined to consider each item separately, wanting to offer it to this grandchild or that. It wasn't hard to imagine scenarios of hurt feelings—the designated receiver not being interested in a given item while somebody else wondered why it hadn't been offered to *them*. Also, I had just been through several years of our younger generation turning their noses up at our offerings; I wanted to protect her from such painful dismissiveness.

We had a lot of furnishings to deal with, and we couldn't take all summer begging the kids to please come collect this or that. Why not go with my mother's lifelong belief in making everything as much fun as possible? The choosing would be like a game and we could have a final party at her house, everyone showing up with pickups and trailers to collect their prizes.

"And since the kids know how to do eBay," I pointed out, "if they want to help clear things out and put them up for sale, I'd say go ahead."

Mistake.

"Oh, no." This horrified her. "I can't imagine anyone in my family doing something like that!"

Deep breath. What to me sounded like efficient redistribution to her clearly looked like crassly cashing in.

When I got home I emailed Madeline for an appointment. Obviously I was heading back into a brand new stress zone. I would once again need help staying centered.

While the story of a middle-aged woman trying to get off of physician-prescribed drugs is going to become increasingly common, it hasn't been told too often yet. The story of a daughter helping her elderly mother move out of her house? You may very well already know the drill.

For starters, though, do not picture my mother helplessly dithering over every old newspaper clipping; she was actually rather decisive, and I'd be surprised if anyone could show me another 87-year-old mother who did more of her own sorting than mine.

So we had that going for us. What we did *not* have was a daughter in the best mental shape. Even on good days, my central nervous system was still whacko, my heart prone to unleashing itself at the slightest hint of conflict. Spiking blood pressure or tachycardia—my brain took charge of choosing which it would be, not me.

When I felt up to it, those hot summer days, I'd drive across town to her house and pack up dishes and weed the cracks in her sidewalks. Clare, after all, would be coming around demanding her usual high standards when we listed the house.

"I'm just not sure what to do about the encyclopedias," my mom would say for the fifth time. "They'll take them down at the used book store, I guess."

"Don't worry, we'll take care of it," I'd say.

"I was thinking I could hire the neighbor boy to take them away."

"We've got this, Mom, don't worry. All you need to do is decide what you want to keep and what you want us to…take some place else."

I had knocked my lights out photographing every last item and writing up an auction-style flyer to be studied by the grandkids, pestering my own kids to speedily forward me their selections. My brother and I had made quick work of the choosing, and I now had my printed-out list of which household was taking what, and I was sorting things into piles and labeling them for efficiency on the day everyone showed up for the dispersal pizza party.

"I'm just surprised no one wanted this painting," Mom said, standing at the bottom of the stairs.

"You said you wanted to take that to the apartment."

"I did?"

I nodded. "I never even took a picture of it."

And later she talked about where in the apartment she planned to put a certain file cabinet.

"But, Mom, you said you didn't want that. I put it on the list and Bob asked for it."

"I never said that."

Oh, dear. I knew I was right. Would rather have been wrong. My mother had remained fairly sharp to this point. I desperately needed that to continue. Evidence to the contrary sent me sinking with dismay.

I remember one day pouring out my anxiety about my mother's memory lapses as Rose Tian inserted her acupuncture needles into my ankles.

She patiently listened, as she always did, and then said, as if this might be some new idea and helpful, "Maybe she's getting Alzheimer's."

Oh, my God. I flashed on yanking out the needles, jumping off the table and running out of there. Instead, I just burst into tears.

This was nuts, I knew, setting myself up against a deadline again, but more than most people suffering through drug withdrawal, especially people coming off benzos, I'd had the luxury of not having to show up at a nine-to-five job or a schedule of university classes. I wasn't in charge of a houseful of kids. Moving my mother was the card I'd drawn and I had to play it.

But trying to keep a bead on the ever-moving target of her preferences seemed to overload my mental wiring, and more than once I was forced to make an abrupt exit from her house. In theory she was grateful for my help, but the reality of me—always exhausted and on edge, unsettlingly contradicting her memory of one thing or another—could not have been much fun. I was not so far gone that I couldn't see this, noting as I did how quick she was to encourage me to—yes, by all means—go home and rest.

In the clearing of her basement, we didn't have time to sit companionably sorting through the family memorabilia, re-telling stories, making guesswork notes of who was who in the old sepia photos. Thus, a half-dozen big green plastic bins went to my house and were now crammed into every available space around the sofas and coffee table in my living room, waiting for me to sort the contents into piles destined for my various cousins.

One of the most satisfying aspects of writing my historical novels has always been the research, but plowing through our own history in my current mental state was a melancholy assignment: Here—sit down and brood over the passing of time, the fleeting nature of our short lives. See if you can sort these pictures without contemplating the fact that most of these people are long dead. As you will be. As everyone you love will be.

On dark days I felt cursed by this, sitting here suffocated by the dusty past, trying to envision some yet unborn individual who might care about all of this in the future. Who would want to read the extremely dry travel journals compiled by my grandfather: **Rest stops were excellent. Very clean**. The vintage travel folders looked eBayable, but would that upset my mother? Was there any historical value in my grandfather's meticulous notations of the price of gas in 1959, or was all this now readily available on the internet anyway?

Might there ever be a great-granddaughter in the future who would be a writer, who might find it fascinating to put back together the pieces of these lives? Would trashing all this be slighting her? Because it's all evidence, and this is why I find it so difficult to throw away the slightest bit of written material. I remember too clearly, in the course of conducting research, the shivering thrills I've experienced at finding a relevant photo with scribbled identification in a historical archive, my gratitude that somebody thought to lodge it there, rather than just take the expedient route to the dump.

Then again, on days when the darkness lifted and I felt surely I was almost well, this pile of memorabilia looked much more benign. Fondly taken childhood portraits—my father was a professional photographer—and shots of family vacations and holiday celebrations seemed evidence that I had been given the sort of childhood that boded well for my ultimate healing. I had been welcomed into the world.

My mother had been incapable of supporting me through this baffling illness of mine, linked as it was to drugs, intractable as it had been to sunny prescriptions for positive thinking. But early on I'd received the gold-standard foundation for a lifetime of solid mental health: as a child I'd been properly cherished.

I was by no means an extravagantly attractive little girl—ask my handsome, Harvard-grad cousin, who once kindly reassured me that the male contingent of his side of the family had come to agree that, at twenty-two, I had actually turned out much better than they had ever expected (!) But my mother had done her best, sympathizing with me that she, too, had wanted Shirley Temple ringlets but, unfortunately, we neither of us had the wonderfully thick curly hair required. Each evening she had dipped a comb in a glass of water set on the coffee table and twisted my thin brown strands into flat coils, fastening them to my scalp with Bobbi pins for the night. The morning results were always disappointing, but it wasn't for her lack of trying.

More than one childhood friend has in later years spontaneously offered up to me memories of genuine envy of my relationship with my mother. A neighbor girl remembers visiting with her own mother, being amazed to find us cozily conferring over sewing patterns and potential shopping trips for fabric. Apparently other mothers could be much more distant than the one with which I'd been blessed.

Mine had always been my biggest fan, marveling at my creativity, pointing out I must have gotten if from my father. (Correct!) She always expressed unending faith that I would somehow come out a winner in whatever I tried. She nurtured resilience in my brain, the very thing I most needed now to hang in there long enough to get well. She had encouraged in me what some call *grit*—a sense of faith in one's own strength to overcome failures, the ability, as the Japanese proverb puts it, to *Fall down seven times, stand up eight.*

Along with my family's memorabilia, I was also helping Herb go through bankers boxes of vintage greeting cards, apparently every single one ever received by anyone in his family. (Never any mystery about his hoarding genes.) His grandmother, whom I adored, often clipped off and saved the charming floral illustrations, perhaps intending them for some future project.

One day I found the cut-off cover of a card featuring a kitty in a yellow basket of red primroses with green leaves, all festooned with a blue bow. I'm sentimental for primary colors, and since I don't like cards with the bossy directive—**Get well!**—this salutation seemed to strike the perfect note of encouragement: **To Hope You're Improving**.

I decided to accept this kindly message from Beyond as intended for me—thanks, Grandma Miles—and taped it up over my computer.

It's still there.

I didn't make it to the last gathering at my mother's house. When the day arrived for pizza and the showing off of the newest babies, I remained in my own backyard with a glass of wine, unaccountably surprised anew, as I was every time, at how systemic the symptoms of pain and fatigue would always be, how shockingly smacked-down I would inevitably feel.

My mother had expressed expectations for how the party would go, outlining little speeches she planned to make with the ritual distribution of certain items, and after exhausting myself getting everything set up, I didn't have it in me for this final wrangling of generations and possessions, couldn't summon the emotional stability to show up and energetically guarantee to make everything nice for her. What if her grandkids didn't come across as suitably grateful? What if she tinkled a glass for attention and nobody shut up to listen?

I tried to explain this to daughter Mary when she sat under the locust tree with me for awhile before going over to the party, but she had disturbingly little to say in response. Obviously, I was boring her. Or, wait. Was this just the gray vapor of paranoia seeping in, distorting my analysis of the words and facial expressions of even the people I loved best in the world? I wondered uneasily if perhaps I had become a subject of discussion at her house. Had it been agreed that encouraging me with questions about my frustrating inability to get well might actually be considered enabling? That I might heal more quickly if people were careful not to let me pay too much attention to myself?

Hey, I knew my story was boring; bored the hell out of me, too.

And I couldn't get in the car and drive away from it.

CHAPTER 31

What a way to live. What an existence. One day I'd be having my morning coffee in my favorite **Make it happen** mug; the next it'd have to be the red and white one Mary gave me: **Keep calm and carry on.**

Nothing illustrated the on-again-off-again, rollercoaster nature of my brain's production of the proper feel-good chemicals than my attitude towards my wardrobe.

On a good day, I could stand before my stuffed closet and simply marvel. Look at all these beautiful new clothes, all these printed silks billowing out. I loved every Johnny Was embroidered blouse, every Sundance dress. Wasn't this amazing? It was like my own personal shopper—talented and knowing—had been cleverly at work while I was out sick, and now, here was a wonderful wardrobe for my new, healthy life, everything perfectly chosen, just for me!

Brilliant, the way I'd optimistically sat at the computer with a glass of wine, credit card at the ready, ordering up the clothes I could picture myself wearing when I was out in the world again. I had Carhartts for working in the woods, Athleta yoga pants and tops for hitting the gym, long velvet skirts and scarves for tribal belly dance class, vintage-look school-marmy outfits I'd worn while lecturing on the background for my historical novels. I even had an unworn, gorgeously beaded dress bought on sale from Peruvian Connection suitable for taking the podium to accept a major award, and a lacy white wedding–style caftan for celebrating an anniversary on the beach in Hawaii. Whatever lay in store, I was ready. I was rooting for myself, even if nobody else was. I was going to get well, dammit, and wear these clothes!

But then, on another day, mind darkened by ever-lingering pain and defeat, the whole stash just looked like so much incriminating evidence of a highly addictive brain struggling to satisfy itself. Who let this woman *do* this? Appalling. Useless excess. Totally delusional. What life of mine would be requiring clothes like this? Not to mention I'd lost the ability to wear a high percentage of these waistbanded skirts about fifteen pounds ago.

Pathetic.

If I'd known what still lay ahead, even at this point—eighteen months off of Oxycodone and ten months off of Xanax—I would have been stocking up, had I been practical, on nothing more than pajamas, a robe, and a bunch of sad, fuzzy socks.

In full meltdown one day, I put in a call to my Ob/Gyn's office in a bid to get my annual exam moved up. I liked Dr. Card; seeing her might be a comfort. The quaver in my voice must have prompted the receptionist to ask just exactly what was going on, and the sound of her sympathy reduced me to a tearful explanation, which I concluded with the lament that I just couldn't believe the clinic didn't seem to have anyone who dealt with prescription drug withdrawal. Doctors got me into this trouble; why couldn't doctors help me out?

Her voice brightened. "Actually, the clinic has just hired a pain specialist who does deal with this. Want me to transfer you right over there?"

Well, of course I did, but naturally, it wouldn't be that simple. I'd need a referral from my PCP. More calls. More waiting while the cheerleadery voice of the clinic, evidently hoping to steer people away from this silly old business of trying to talk on the phone to other actual humans, repeatedly exhorted me to "Google us today and feel better faster!"

Imagine how I was answering that recording as I paced my kitchen.

"Google us today and feel better faster!"

Especially on the fourth or fifth loop.

Several weeks of hoop jumping for insurance purposes ensued, during which I was assured Dr. Nash was studying my files to make sure he could help me. When I told my long-standing, pre-surgery physical therapist about this, she sounded a warning.

"Are you sure he's right for you? He had an article in the paper a while back—you know, thanks for welcoming me to Corvallis—and it sounded like he was a lot more into prescribing opioids than in getting people off of them." She'd been struck by his lack of mention of any alternative therapies for pain such as acupuncture or physical therapy.

This gave me pause, and since Dr. Nash's office wasn't phoning me back about an appointment, I let it slide. To be stalled so long did not bode well, and when they finally did call with the offer of an appointment, I hesitated.

"Could I ask you guys a question first?" I explained the doubts that had been raised. I wasn't actually a pain patient. I had long been completely off the painkilling pills and mainly just needed reassurance from someone with experience in weaning people off these drugs that I hadn't missed anything and was on the right track.

"You know," she said, "That's a very good question." She promised to look into it and get back to me.

When somebody finally called back a week or two later, I repeated my concern.

"Oh, yes," the voice on the phone reassured me, "Dr. Nash is very familiar with the insurance code on your file."

I booked what was to be a forty-minute consultation and dutifully filled out the lengthy intake forms which were mailed to me, explaining that I was suffering from post-acute withdrawal syndrome.

"Any bets what he'll say?" I asked Herb on the drive across town to the clinic that summer morning. I wanted my husband with me, and in order to take the soonest offered appointment, we'd had to cancel our usual morning play date with our little grandson. Bummer for Herb. I knew who was more fun to be with, and it wasn't me.

"No idea," Herb said, "but can I make one suggestion? I'd be careful talking about feeling suicidal if you don't want to be triggering all sorts of drastic interventions."

We'd had this discussion so many times. I completely understood his concern. It's just that I'd always felt that using the term suicidal ideation was the only way to convey the depths of my distress.

"If you have to," Herb went on, "maybe you could emphasize that you're a strong person and you feel confident you'd never do that."

I looked at my husband, who was keeping his eyes on Third Street through downtown. Probably he'd like for me to be giving this reassurance more often for *his* benefit too.

"Well, I'm fine today," I promised.

Walking into this brand new, pastel-decorated wing of the clinic, I was glad and grateful that my long-awaited appointment had landed on a day randomly selected by my brain to be one where I would feel myself on an even keel.

At least I would start out that way. Sitting in the waiting room, I tried to breathe evenly, taking in the new carpet smell as the time passed. Why were we having to wait? This had to be the doctor's first appointment of the day. You knew he wasn't doing emergency surgery.

"Take it easy," Herb whispered, wanting to see me stay calm. "Remember—this may be his first chance to study those papers you handed in."

Maybe that was it. I'd just now given them to the woman at the desk. Nervously, I kept popping out to the restroom. At least there weren't any cameras in there. That I knew of, anyway.

Finally a nurse came out to fetch us.

"Oh, I'm sorry," she said when Herb got up to follow me. "Dr. Nash insists on seeing patients alone."

Herb frowned. "Why's that?"

"It's just the way he wants to do it. She can ask him if you can come in."

I made distressed eyes at Herb and followed her to get weighed and measured.

In the exam room, she wrapped the blood pressure monitor around my arm and started pumping up the dial.

"I'm sure that made it go up," I said, "not letting my husband in."

Yep. Over the past months my blood pressure had normalized to where I'd been able to wean off the meds, but this sort of thing could still make it spike.

I sat alone for fifteen minutes more until Dr. Nash finally came in and introduced himself. Okay, so I finally had my white coat. Over a pink oxford shirt.

"Um, I'd really like to have my husband with me for this."

"Why? You're a grownup."

I blinked. Excuse me? Grownups don't need support?

"I wanted him to hear what you have to say, too. We booked this forty-minute consult and he didn't even bring his Kindle." I was thinking that if Herb couldn't be with me, I'd have driven myself, and he could have stayed home and had fun with Noley.

"I don't like to have the spouse in the room when I'm dealing with pain patients wanting prescriptions."

"But I'm not a pain patient."

"What do you mean?" He tapped a line on my chart. "Says right here your primary care doctor sent you to me for lower back pain."

I glanced at the scribbled line. "I never told her that."

He grunted. "So, just how long have you been seeing this Dr. Miller?"

"Only a few years," I said. "She hasn't known me as long as all the doctors I had who retired."

Looking back, all I can think is, oh my God—lamb to the slaughter. While I was busy thinking I was supposed to be apologizing to this man for having myself referred by somebody who hadn't actually delivered me as a baby (the main clinic building was named Asbury, for the doctor who had), removed the sewing needle from my knee five decades ago, or delivered my own three babies, he was already way down another road entirely. I think he was set to pounce on me as a doctor shopper, a drug-seeking addict never seeing any given doctor more than a time or two.

"You need to go right back to her," he said, startlingly angry all of a sudden. "You ask her why she did this."

Seriously? My long-awaited consultation had instantly turned into an office politics dispute?

"But I never lied about anything. I'm suffering from post-acute withdrawal syndrome. That's what I told your receptionist. That's what I wrote on those papers you had me fill out."

Obviously he hadn't bothered to read a single word.

"If you've got post-acute withdrawal syndrome, you need to be put on Suboxone."

Suboxone? He was talking about the drug they dispense at rehab clinics?

"Okay, I really need my husband to be hearing this."

"Oh, all right." Dr. Pain Management made no effort to hide his exasperation. "You go get him."

He disappeared, apparently having more important things to do than wait the sixty seconds this required. Herb and I sat waiting another ten minutes before he reappeared. Either my pulse was racing or my blood pressure was spiking. I felt awful.

When he came back in, I began my story, starting with the surgery, explaining how I'd come to be taking so much Oxycodone, how I'd done a rapid taper over the course of three weeks.

"And then, a couple of weeks after that, I had my first window, but of course that was just the first and right after that—"

"Wait a minute. What do you mean when you say, 'a window?'"

"You know, when you feel well for awhile." This was common parlance on all the addiction and withdrawal sites on the internet, but he looked blank.

I glanced at Herb. So much for worrying about alarming this guy with admissions of feeling suicidal.

I tried to pick up with my story, but Dr. Nash acted like he'd already heard enough. My narrative was irrelevant. It seemed I wasn't a person he could help, or, more importantly, somebody he should be *expected* to help.

"What I want to know," he said, "is why you're walking in here so mad at *me?*"

Helplessly, I looked at Herb.

"She's really had a lot of bad experiences with doctors lately," Herb said. "I'm afraid you're getting the brunt of that."

Oh, my God. My husband was *apologizing* for *me?* And for what?

"Well, I keep reading I should seek medical help," I said, "and I've tried, but it doesn't seem like there's any help for somebody like me."

"Well, I'm certainly no addictionologist."

"I know that. But you seemed like the closest thing the clinic had. I was just hoping for some stories about people like me who've gotten well. Some reassurance."

"Reassurance?" He snorted. "Look at you. You're sitting here just full of vitriol and anger."

I looked past him to Herb. "Are you *hearing* this?" Why was he just sitting there? Why had he actually apologized for me like I was some kind of pouty little girl best dealt with by a bit of humoring? Looking back, in his defense, he'd been as blindsided as I had by this doctor's demeanor. He'd been gearing up to defend me from commitment to a mental institution, not anticipating the need for snappy comebacks to garden-variety insults.

I do think this moment, though, burned into my memory, might qualify as traumatizing. Over a full year later I would have a nightmare of being attacked by a rabid sheep, which knocked me down, wrapped itself around me and started gnawing on my shoulder as Herb calmly watched. "Aren't you going to stop it?" I cried. "Aren't you going to defend me?" Dream husband just shrugged. "I figured you were just getting what you deserved."

Still, I was ultimately grateful for Herb's witness that day. Would he have believed me when I quoted this doctor if he hadn't heard it himself? *Vitriol.* What a word. Who even uses it in conversation?

Now I remembered to tell Dr. Nash I'd also been on Xanax. He'd cut off my story before I got to that part.

"So which do you think is giving you withdrawal symptoms?" he asked.

"Well, probably both."

"Exactly." He rolled his eyes.

Seriously? I'd gone off both opioids and benzos just as soon as anybody hinted I ought to. I'd never relapsed. And now the fact that I was still unaccountably suffering somehow made me the most annoying patient ever to walk in this man's office? If this is how he treated me, I just couldn't imagine his approach to the poor souls in physical pain, approaching him on bended knee in hopes of a refill of their Vicodin.

Dr. Nash started lecturing about the opioid epidemic. "All those kids hooked on heroin over there in Lebanon and Sweet Home? They all got started on prescriptions drugs."

"I know," I said. "I'm writing a book about it."

This seemed to go right past him. He started talking about 12-step programs and how the best experts now feel that it's absolutely necessarily to give people replacement treatment in the form of Suboxone in order to prevent relapse.

"But I'm not relapsing," I said. "I haven't taken Oxycodone for nineteen months. I don't want to be on another drug I'll just have to worry about getting off of." Hadn't he read all the stories from people claiming they simply couldn't kick Suboxone?

"You shouldn't even be here," he said. "You should be seeing an addictionologist."

"I did go see Susan Spaulding last fall."

He snorted. "She's a flake. Just a primary care physician with a Suboxone license." This in a derisive, sing-song tone. "And she doesn't wear shoes!"

Having already heard the barefoot bit from me, Herb smirked. "Looks like you've got the dress code down a little better than she does."

Yeah, great—these guys having a laugh over this. At least Susan Spaulding had been kind. At least she'd offered some respect for my discipline in getting off the narcotics so rapidly. I regret now not defending her to Dr. Nash, but I couldn't even seem to defend myself here. And this guy wasn't hearing anything I was saying anyway. Sorry, Susan.

But I hated thinking this had all been a waste. Making one more grab at a crumb of comfort, I pleaded, "Can't you just tell me how long it usually takes to get better?"

"No," he said, "I can't. You just don't want to face the reality that you have two choices here. You either need to go on Suboxone or join a 12-step program."

That's when I gave up. This visit had not had anything to do with me or my specific case from the minute I'd been separated from my husband in the waiting room. I sank back into my corner, stunned and beaten, while the doctor railed to Herb, man to man, about the inadequacies of the medical system and how there was no insurance money in addiction treatment. He even managed to drag Obama's name into the blame game.

I burst into tears the minute we left the exam room, and snagged a tissue in the waiting room on the way out. I will always wonder if the people I passed in the lineup of chairs figured I was upset at not being given the narcotics I'd been seeking.

I cried furiously all the way home, but then I stopped. Because this wasn't dopamine depletion depression, this was raw outrage at having patiently waited for this appointment in hopes of compassion, only to get—and these were Herb's words, not mine—condescension, sarcasm, and abuse.

Too bad he hadn't said those words straight to the guy's face.

Too bad for this abuse we would be getting a bill.

I stopped crying, came up to my office and wrote down, while they were fresh, this medical professional's every appalling word.

I want to be fair, though. Maybe he was just having a bad day? After belatedly finding some terrible on-line reviews for this man, however, it seems clear if it was a bad day, it was definitely not his first.

So let's just say it's entirely possible he is perfectly decent to his cat.

CHAPTER 32

I took it hard when I saw Dr. Leman's obituary in the local paper. I hadn't seen him since that day at the library nearly two years before. Hadn't seen anyone really, stuck at home as I'd been. He, in contrast, had apparently been out and about until the end. My mother heard he'd been at a party just a few days before his death. People were saying that his embraces had seemed particularly lingering and heartfelt recently though, as if perhaps he sensed any goodbye might be the final one.

When you reach a certain age and your family has lived in the same town since your grandparents met there in college, you find yourself in line for potential attendance at a lot of funerals. I'd been to plenty over the years, but had missed almost all that had come up since my surgery.

I was feeling stable when the date for Dr. Leman's service arrived, however, and for this man we had both so much admired, there was no question—my mother and I would go.

We were clearly not alone in our high regard for him; the Unitarian Church was packed. I saw my original ob/gyn, Tom Hart, along with other staff from the clinic I recognized. I shifted on the back pew to make room for John Berry, the wonderful pediatrician who had reassured me about my ability to nurse my twins. The stories of his kindness to our Cambodian friends when they first arrived in town found their way into the character of Jonathan's physician father in my novel, *Children of the River.*

And then I spotted the anesthesiologist who'd been summoned from bed on the cold January night my water broke, heralding the twins. Remembering our brief and needlessly unpleasant encounter before he got that needle stuck into my back, I was struck anew at how indelibly every interaction with these men—and yes, they were all men—had been inked upon my brain.

I would be very surprised if anyone had a bad memory involving Dr. Leman, however, and if they'd opened the mike, we'd have been there until the following morning. The remembrances of his invited eulogists were all of his loving kindness to his patients, his colleagues, his friends, and his family. Dr. Clifford Hall told a story of finding him sitting at the bed of a homeless man, just to spare this stranger from dying alone.

It was agreed: the world would be a poorer place without him, but a better place for his having been here. "The Conscience of the Corvallis Clinic," he had been called over the years. Much was made of his campaign to steer Corvallis toward being smoke-free. Over and over he'd tried to quit smoking himself, finally succeeding only after his third or fourth attempt. He understood the difficulty of addiction, how hard it is to go through the illness of withdrawal and resist the quick fix of one more cigarette.

He'd have understood about doctor-caused addiction. He'd have seen what we're coming up against with both benzo and opioid withdrawal in the population. If his race hadn't been run, I could picture him taking on the whole mess as a public health issue, just as he'd taken on the problem of smoking. He'd have been advocating for patients who needed compassionate treatment, not incarceration.

Sitting there, gazing up at the wooden ceiling beams as Dr. Leman's friends played the classical music he loved, it hit me. In my desperate casting call for a figure of white-coated kindness, look who had shown up. Surely his healing spirit had not expired just because he was gone. Even dead he was a better candidate for my purposes than any of the live doctors I had encountered recently. Next time I fell into the black hole, I would simply channel from him the encouragement I needed. Dr. Leman understood about hope. He even gave his daughter that name. No trick at all to hear him delivering these lines.

You hang in there.

You're going to be fine.

You're strong and brave, and if other people have made it through this, you can too.

You're almost well, so don't you dare think of giving up the fight now.

Remember that I'm rooting for you.

I went home and taped to my mirror the funeral program featuring his benevolent countenance.

It's still there.

CHAPTER 33

———————◄

I felt great all Labor Day weekend at Neskowin, where both sons joined us. The best part was watching Miles be the gung-ho, goofy, sand-shoveling daddy for darling Noley, Miles who at the age of seven had memorably pouted on our first day of possession: "Do we have to come here a lot?"

After a long run of years where it seemed the kids would always be too busy with soccer or their college lives to spend time with us at the beach, now here they were, totally into it. Everything was turning out as we'd always hoped, and once again the future looked promising.

Driving home with Herb through the forested Van Duzer corridor, I was practically high. I remembered how I'd lamented the timing of the baby, how I'd feared everything would be spoiled if I couldn't be one hundred percent well by his birth. Good thing I wasn't in charge of arranging things, because now Nolan's timing seemed perfect. For Herb, becoming a grandfather had put a new spring in his step, as if taking on this role that came only with age had actually made him feel younger.

And as for me, when you are trying to be all about living in the *now*, I swear, there is nothing better than the precious moments you get with a baby. Especially in the early months, the warm weight of that child in my arms, the inhaling of his special baby scent was the best medicine ever. I'd been so down on myself for so long, I'd been so convinced I'd do everything wrong as a grandma; how affirming to find that—hey—at our house at least, amazing as Herb was as a grandfather, it was *me* who had the pillowy anatomy to hold the baby in the way that most comforted him. I'd mothered three babies; I knew how to manage this gig.

Even better now, though, I was no longer the ambitious young woman who just kept trying to get things *done*. Rock the babies? Great, but who was going to get the laundry going? Clean up the kitchen? Write that book? Now I understood how fleeting was the blissful time when a baby wanted only to be held, and nothing else I might be doing seemed more compelling than simply sitting in the rocker with him while he napped, whispering the story to him of how much he was loved and how glad we all were that he had arrived. I had always credited my constant stream of commentary to his daddy with helping him turn out to be the precociously verbal little whippersnapper that he was, and I figured I'd try the same technique on his son.

As we swooped into view of the Cascades to the east, I turned to Herb.

"I really feel like I'm on the verge of living the very best years of my life."

Three hours later, I was down in the pit again.

The first nudge toward the black hole was finding in the accumulated mail at home the insurance statement showing that despite all the hoop jumping for pre-approval, Regence Blue Cross Blue Shield would not cover my visit to Dr. Nash, the pain specialist, or even put the charges toward my deductible. No surprise, but annoying, the reminder that they would have nothing to do with recovery from addiction. So what if you'd been addicted by the very doctors whose services they *had* covered.

I held out a glimmer of hope that the clinic would have taken notice of the immediate letter of protest over this nightmare of a visit I'd sent them, and have the good grace not to charge me. No such luck. Later that day, in a fresh batch of mail, here came the bill: $287.

"I'm not paying," I said to Herb.

"Well, wait a minute here...."

"No, I've already made up my mind. I am not paying this bill."

"We need to think about this, though. We don't want the clinic mad at us."

I stared at him. "You're worried about *them* being mad at *us*?"

"You should be thinking about the rest of the family. What if they kick everybody out? I don't want to have to find a new doctor."

"I'm not afraid of the clinic. They should be afraid of me! I'm pretty damned sure I could make a case for more than two hundred and eighty-seven dollars worth of pain and suffering at the hands of that jerk. They're lucky I'm not suing *them!*"

I went up to my office and knocked out a letter to the clinic's finance department, explaining why I would not be paying. I included a copy of my first letter of protest. My connection with the Corvallis Clinic went back almost to its 1949 inception, my birth following it by just two years. I'd racked up a lifetime of charges and never before not paid, but I would not be paying this bill now.

"It feels like no one sticks up for me," I told Madeline at our next session. "And I've always stuck up for everybody else."

On the medical front, I'd advocated for my mom, my kids, and each time Herb got wheeled into an operating room—there'd been several—I was always following his gurney, informing anybody in scrubs who'd listen that he had a strong gag reflex and had actually thrown up under anesthetic one time, a very dangerous situation. Would they please watch this very closely? And keep in mind that this man they're cutting open is beloved by so many who count on him?

More than once I'd hauled him to the doctor and effectively sped up his cure for this or that, but he never similarly took charge for me. He always expected me to make the decision. It never mattered how sick and vulnerable my state, how compromised my cognitive capacity, he always insisted on relying on me to tell him what to do.

This had been the story our entire marriage, it seemed to me, and now, when I was down in the pit and depressed to death, the toxic ruminations over this could steadily feed a long hard crying session.

I needed him to say *Screw the clinic, I've got your back*.

Madeline listened to all this and then said, in effect: *Give it up*.

"You're the one who's different," she said. "You're the one willing to fight. Herb's reaction is pretty much what most people do."

"Yeah?"

"Sure. Most people avoid confrontation. I hear all sorts of stories about people unhappy with their doctors, but everybody's got reasons why they're scared to make waves. You're pretty much at the far end of the spectrum for speaking up."

A few weeks later I got a call from the clinic's finance department. A friendly woman wanted to let me know that the charges for my visit with Dr. Nash had somehow been dropped. She sounded a bit mystified.

"It seems to be something about not being able to find a proper insurance code for your visit."

I laughed. "Okay, if that's how they want to do it." I explained why this was absolutely the correct course on their part. She seemed interested. Maybe the people in billing aren't quite so locked in to the protocol of defending a colleague no matter how bad he messes up.

"They better start calling it Post Acute Withdrawal Syndrome Due to Addiction by a Physician's Prescription," I told the finance woman. "I think you're going to be seeing more of this coming through in the future."

My sparkly little mother had amazed everyone in the apartment tour group by making it, cane in hand, all the way up three flights of roughed-in steps to the top floor.

Wow. The two of us looked at each other, wide-eyed. The view from her apartment was going to be stunning—to the east, the Willamette River and the Cascades in the distance and to the west, the historic Benton County Courthouse and iconic Marys Peak.

I ordered a special bench arrangement for the west entry deck—two wooden chairs attached to a drink table and angled slightly toward each other. Perfect for my sociable mother. She'd waste no time snagging Happy Hour company to watch the sunsets.

Knowing she would eschew anything that smacked of "handicapped," I ran around lining up attractive bathtub grab bars which the management promised they'd be happy to install. I was so pleased when they asked me if I thought my mother would appreciate having her cabinets set slightly lower. Absolutely, I wrote back, ridiculously tickled to feel how well I was handling all of this.

Ha! I may have had a grasp of the concept of feng shui, but I knew nothing of leasing apartments, especially a unit in a building still under construction. The management kept insisting that move-in date was still September 1st, even as it was clear to anyone watching the workers on scaffolding that the building was not going to be ready for occupancy for several more weeks.

Our plan had been to move Mom to the apartment, and only then swiftly clean and stage her house for the market. When the management finally admitted the apartment occupancy date would be postponed, we were forced to Plan B, which meant putting the house on the market while she was still living there. Not ideal, but we couldn't afford to be pushing our market date into the rainy season. The gray gloom of winter in Oregon never made any property look more appealing.

My mother's voice on the phone that September Day sounded like death—low, gravelly, from the grave.

"What's my apartment number?" No greeting. No preamble. Just this question.

"It's 407," I said.

"They're telling me it's 405. I went down to the office to see what I could find out about the move-in date and they say they have me in 405."

"Well, 405 was the original one we reserved, but after the tour, we switched it to 407, remember? I dropped those grab bars off marked unit 407."

"And I already had my return address labels with the sailboats printed with the number 407."

"Okay, I'll talk to them, Mom. We'll get this straightened out."

Looking back at this tempest in a teapot, I remember how, that day, it seemed to me more like a tidal wave. Later my mother explained that the gravity in her voice had been solely out of concern for the way she feared I might flip out, which of course makes complete sense, the unbearably edgy way I was forever reacting to everything. What I heard in her voice, though, sounded like grave disappointment. I had let my mother down. I had knocked my lights out trying to properly manage this business and now somehow I'd blown it. Never mind that all my emails (I checked) had included the correctly changed unit number, I had made promises to her I couldn't now keep. Would she be getting the lowered cabinets? Had the designer grab bars I'd bought been installed in somebody else's unit?

I thought I'd been doing so well. I'd been experiencing flashes of enjoyment and satisfaction from thinking I knew how to manage things.

But no, what an idiot; I'd blown it.

I see now how poorly my brain was still functioning, how low were my reserves in handling stress. Not to mention the ludicrousness of thinking I could herd the batch of cats the apartment management team turned out to be, people who didn't know themselves what was going on or what would happen next.

The Willamette Valley had been rainless for weeks, and in a dry field on the north side of town, a couple of teenagers smoking dope dared each other to toss a match. The hillside was soon consumed in flames that flared alarmingly close to nearby houses.

My brain felt like that field, dry and brittle, and now somebody had tossed a match.

After my mother's call, I fell on my carpeted sewing room floor, curled up in a ball and started crying. I couldn't do this. I shouldn't be *trying* to do it. My brain was so sickly fragile. I knew better than to set myself up for stress and yet here I was, smacked down with the news one more time: **You are not in control.**

I heard Herb bringing the baby up the stairs.

Oh, for God's sake. "No, take him away."

"I thought he might cheer you up."

"Herb, I do not want him to see me this way." I didn't want the briefest memory of me like this burned into his bright little brain. I wanted to be the grandma who swept him up and danced him around the house to "Who's My Pretty Baby?"

"Well, I don't want to leave you alone like this."

"I know," I said, hiding my face, "but it's okay. Just let me cry."

In the moving of my mother, I was not trying for martyrdom. When my brother offered to come up from Eugene for a day and help Mom clear things out, I was grateful. A cleaning crew was scheduled to do a top-to-bottom just before the house went on the market, my bid for avoiding stress, not inviting it.

And yet, on the last day before sending my mother off to her Yachats beach cabin and officially turning the place over to Clare, I walked into my mother's house post-cleaning and couldn't stop myself from trying to do something about the handsome brick wall in the kitchen. Clearly the cleaners hadn't touched it. I considered it the kitchen's best feature. It wouldn't do to have grease spots on it. Clare certainly wouldn't approve.

Before long I was huffing and puffing, scrubbing away, making the whole thing worse by apparently using the wrong cleanser. Looking satisfyingly clean while still wet, the minute a patch dried, the white streaks revealed the damage I was doing. Oh, shit. So stupid. I'd just wanted to make this one little thing better and now it looked awful.

Herb was moving through at his usual languid pace, hanging potted green houseplants, filling the half-barrel planter on the front porch with russet mums. Mom had unaccountably decided this would be a good time to give her dust pan a thorough scrubbing at the kitchen sink. They both tried to assure me the bricks didn't matter.

Didn't matter? On what HGTV house-staging show would this not matter? Didn't they have eyes? Couldn't they see how horrible it looked? I kept going over the same areas, hoping for a better outcome, not getting it, trying the same thing again—the very definition of insanity. After an hour or two, I was weepy with fatigue, melting down. I flashed back to the bathroom floor at the Jackson Avenue bungalow, how I hadn't wanted to flip out in earshot of Eleanor next door. I couldn't go that route in front of my mother either. *Xanax*, I was thinking. *Now* is when I'd want to be popping a tab.

Anything worth doing at all is worth doing well—an admonition I heard repeatedly as a child. I'm sure my mother never intended to cripple me with perfectionism, though. She was probably thinking along the lines of *Don't be a slacker*. And in any case, she never expected me to take everything she said so seriously. "For heaven's sakes," has been her response every time in later years when I've quoted her, "if I'd known you were paying such close attention, I'd have been more careful with what I said!"

Now, in the kitchen where she'd been cooking for nearly fifty years and I was on the verge of freaking out entirely, she said, "I wish you weren't having to do this." Too bad we were past the point where she could have enforced some of the rules that had actually worked rather well when I was a child. If I got frustrated over a sewing project—tangled thread, a pattern piece cut in error—she made me quit and come back to it when I'd calmed down. Rather clever, actually, because I learned that if I did actually want to continue, I couldn't afford the luxury of histrionics. Likewise, when my brother and I were learning to water ski, we got three chances to yell hit it! and then "get up." We'd both been frequently reminded that *If at first you don't succeed,* you should *try, try again,* yes, but my parents also held to the caveat of acknowledging the diminishing returns once the point of physical exhaustion had been reached.

Unfortunately, this cleaning job was not something I could just try, try again later. I couldn't calm down and come back next week. It was now or never.

"I'm just sorry you're having to work so hard," Mom said. "And doing my house, it isn't like when you worked on Will's Portland house and got to stay in a nice hotel and go out to eat."

I froze, scrub brush upheld, soapy splats pinging to the soaked newspapers covering the floor. That's how she saw last year's House-Rehab-During-Drug-Withdrawal Hell? That obviously a hotel and a daily restaurant dinner must have made it a really fun party?

Moving is terribly stressful for an older person, and I'd been given plenty of advice on the importance of my remaining sensitive to this fact, in certain cases from people who had somehow managed to avoid such involvement with their own mothers entirely.

But, okay, got it.

When I was finally able to force myself to give up on the bricks, I tried to gently steer my mother into making the decisions that were hers alone—what to keep/what to toss. I sat with her and went through a box of old framed photos, disassembling them and putting unwanted frames in a giveaway box.

We had a deadline now. Looking back, I can see that my brain had me fired up beyond the necessary. I could have just thrown that box of pictures in the garage with the rest of the stuff that would either go to the apartment or be sorted later, but I was still trying to adhere to the HGTV rule of having all clutter removed from the premises before that first open house. Besides, the way I saw it, people who always advocated relaxing, lightening up and taking it easy never made it to the finish line. Not without us ridiculously uptight people coming along and picking up the pieces.

I encouraged my mom to go through her second closet of clothes and went downstairs to check out the rec room. Great, cobwebs all over the ceiling. I flailed away with a broom. I thought we'd told that cleaning crew we'd pay for the most thorough job possible; now it looked like they'd done their three hours or whatever and called it quits.

By law we'd had to have the fireplace insert removed, and although the used bricks were attractive, gouge marks had been left in the blackened ones around the firebox. I sat on the hearth and reached in for some remaining chunks of charcoal, hoping to manage a quick artistic fix, coloring in the light orange scratches.

Scrabbling around in there, blackening my hands, I thought, *Oh my God, look—I've turned into Cinderella.*

"Hey, come here," Herb called from the bottom of the stairs.

"What," I said. "I'm all ashy."

"Well, this is worth it," he promised.

At the bottom of the stairs I looked up and saw my mother modeling her most recent wedding gown, a floor-length concoction of beaded chiffon in a flattering shade of champagne.

She smiled and executed a small twirl. "I just had to stop and try this on."

She had been a beautiful bride at seventy-five for my Prince Charming of a step-father and now, over a decade later, she could still rock that dress.

"You look gorgeous," I said, and it was true.

CHAPTER 34

Lovely, to be well enough that Sunday in September that we could risk getting in the truck to go put in a day of woods work at one of our coast range forest properties—limbing trees, fighting back Scotch broom. This is what I'd so sorely missed all these months.

We each worked separately that morning, then unfolded our beat-up lawn chairs on the bridge over Kitten Creek for our picnic lunch together.

I was delighted to find that naturally, even in my absence, the Doug fir and hemlock we'd planted here had continued to grow. My little pruning job made no huge difference in the great scheme of the forest. It was just my excuse to be out there, availing myself of the opportunity for what it turns out the Japanese actually have a name—shinrin-yoku—forest bathing. As I worked, I took in the scent of the sap released from the lopped-off branches and the sun-warmed smell of the already fallen needles baking on the late summer duff. The air itself seemed medicinal. Healing.

Everything seemed perfect. I felt fine.

But then, at day's end, just as we were driving the pick-up down the gravel road, it hit: my chest seized up.

Herb stopped the truck, hustled around to my side, yanked open the door and cranked down the seat. I lay back and, out of habit, checked my watch. We knew the drill. I tried to breathe calmly. He stroked my arms.

"I don't know why it's always so scary," I whimpered.

"Shh. It's just the chemicals."

Cortisol, adrenaline, whatever it took to give you that dreadful rush of darkest doom pouring coldly through your veins. We'd puzzled over this so many times. Didn't people get panic attacks at unusually stressful times? These always hit when I was feeling particularly good, once even while I was holding the baby. Over the previous winter I'd had a six-month stretch without any, but recently I'd been taken by surprise like this about once a month.

"I want. To stop. Having these." Because every damned time it scared me to death, the way the pain radiated up to my right jaw, a symptom they always list in the of warning signs of a "cardiac event."

"Hang on," Herb murmured. He'd gotten so good at this. "It won't last much longer."

I nodded, holding tight to his calloused, work-worn hands, those hands that had hung onto me through so much. *Breathe deep….breathe deep…*

And then, slowly, the cramp eased up. I took an even deeper breath, released it like a yoga class exhalation. I looked at my watch.

"Five minutes."

"Well, see? You're getting better."

Yeah, great. Five minutes is a long time when you feel like you're having a heart attack. Seriously, this business had gotten old a whole year ago.

We cranked my seat up, buckled ourselves back in, and drove down to find dinner in some coastal café where nobody would look twice at our dirt-smacked-off-the-best-we-could work clothes.

A few days later my physical therapist listened to my recounting of this recent spate of attacks and suggested a psychologist in Eugene who was using a new technique called neurofeedback. Clearly something was still wonky in my central nervous system. Maybe he could help.

I Googled the concept and decided to give it a shot. It sounded a bit like biofeedback, where you'd learn to control your brain functions with your own thought processes. I thought I'd been doing a decent job of enduring these chest cramping episodes without actually panicking, but was I missing something? If I could be taught to actually *prevent* a recurrence, that would be a very good thing indeed.

The Eugene offices of Dr. Glen Tibbets, Ph.D. offered a twenty-session package.

Although I knew I should be taking the relaxed, zen-like approach to the timeline of my healing, the idea of a treatment where I could be more proactive had an undeniable appeal to my latent A-Type side.

After I scheduled my consultation appointment I received, by email, a slew of intake attachments with a lengthy explanation: **They are very important to the success of your first visit with Dr. Tibbets. Please return all forms at least two business days prior to the appointment.**

Am I supposed to fill out only the forms that are relevant? I wrote back. **Surely not all of these.**

Dr. Tibbets would like you to fill out all of the forms. Even the ones that may seem irrelevant can provide useful information.

Seriously? But I wasn't ADD and it wasn't depression. It was drug withdrawal.

Every little detail is a clue for the doctor, the secretary insisted in reply. **I know it's a pain but it is very useful.**

Okay, thanks for the explanations, I wrote back. **I'll get right on it and do my best. But I'm tired of writing out my story for doctors and then not having them read it. Can you promise me Dr. Tibbets doesn't operate this way?** Then I deleted the last two sentences. No need to go into this with a chip on my shoulder. This particular guy had done nothing yet to deserve my insulting suspicions. He shouldn't have to pay for the bad manners of Dr. Pain Management.

I spent three full hours filling out the twenty-five pages. Herb's input was required on a couple of sections. Apparently people with mental issues can't always be trusted to accurately self-report. Since my story would not conveniently compress itself into boxes for checking off, and didn't lend itself to the assigning of numbers to moods, I ended up writing a cover letter, concluding with how much I was looking forward to learning if his techniques could help me.

"Even though those papers were a pain," I told Herb as we took the tight curve on 99W driving to Eugene a week later, "I'm glad now. It's a relief to know I won't have to sit there and tell this whole story again. It'll be nice to walk in and talk to somebody who's actually studied my case."

Although I'd been tempted to mark **Not Applicable** on at least half of the twenty-five pages, I'd tried to give useful information. I'd appreciated the chance to let this doctor know me as an individual.

The mandatory ADD form asked if I'd ever had special programs set up for me in school. **Yes,** I wrote, halfway smart-ass, **but mine were because I was too far ahead.**

What was my highest level of education and what was my grade point average? **Don't remember the grades,** I wrote, **but they must have been good because I graduated Phi Beta Kappa.** Ha! Phi Beta Crappa, Herb always joked. It had been years after college before I realized this designation meant anything to anybody, but now I was glad for this bit of evidence to substantiate my claim that I actually had a mind worthy of retrieval.

One page asked me to check off all instances of abuse I had been subjected to as a child, followed by all the abuses of my mother I may have witnessed. I quickly ticked off **never never never** to everything. At the bottom I was asked what I considered my greatest strength.

My resilience, I wrote, **with which I'm no doubt blessed due to the fact that I was able to check "no" to everything above.**

In the space for listing recent stressful events, I'd written of being in the midst of moving my mother out of her house, knowing that was one of those recognizable life events that earned you points on the stress scale.

In truth, though, by the time we were driving to Eugene that autumn day, I was feeling quite calm about at least that episode in my life. No, my mother didn't get the apartment we thought she would. But here's the thing: *it did not matter.* She got the one I originally designated and it was fine. Actually none of the apartments had been finished with custom-lowered cabinets, and likewise, no problem with her elegant grab bars being installed in the wrong apartment—they hadn't even gotten around to doing that anyway!

Our plan in sending her to the Yachats beach cabin when the house went on the market worked out beautifully; we'd succeeded in finding the buyer before she even came home at the end of the week. Through hints to Clare, we managed to obtain from the buyer a lovely letter praising the house and promising years of family Thanksgivings to be held there—just the words Mom would want to hear to make this transition easier.

"So remind me," Herb said, keeping his eyes on the road. "What is it you want from me in this visit?"

"Well, if I get off track, remember that I'm just there for this first visit to try to figure out if his program can help me. Remind me that we're trying to find out if he's had patients like me and had success with them."

A sign at the building housing various therapists directed us to go around a walkway to the side for Dr. Tibbets office. There, another sign directed us to go back the way we'd come.

Herb and I looked at each other. We didn't have to say it. Not promising. Too Alice-in-Wonderland.

A few minutes later we were ushered back into the doctor's office and the two of us took seats facing him.

He looked expectantly at us, a small smile in place. "Do you have some paperwork for me?"

"Uh...I sent it in."

"Oh, okay." The doctor patted around at papers on his desk.

My heart sank. I looked at Herb. *Tell me this isn't happening.*

"Well, let me go see." The doctor went out to the reception area.

Well, shit. Even if they found it, this meant he hadn't given it the thorough studying promised.

He came back in. "No," he said pleasantly, "they don't have it."

I could have burst into tears right there. "I mailed it last week. In plenty of time."

"Oh, you *mailed* it." As if the method of transmission mattered. The fact was, they didn't have it and clearly, he hadn't noticed until this very minute.

"I wonder if you sent it to our old address." He smiled. "The post office isn't very good about forwarding things."

I couldn't believe this. At the same time, I could. For a Phi Beta Crappa I'm a ridiculously slow learner. Whatever made me imagine for one minute this scene would go the way I'd mentally written it?

He sat there looking at me, waiting.

"So I'm supposed to just start telling you everything I wrote down?"

He gave a little shrug. Like, did I have a better plan?

A great wave of weariness washed over me. What was the point of boring myself (and Herb) with the details spoken aloud all over again? I didn't see how I was going to be able to muster any faith in this guy if this is how he operated.

I sighed, tried to gather myself, and started telling my story.

"Anything else?" he asked after awhile.

I talked some more.

"Anything else?

This was a long and twisted story. I could have gone on for hours.

"Anything else?"

Finally, I said, "Isn't this enough?"

Okay, sure, he was trying to make me feel I'd been heard. He didn't want to be accused of not letting me have my say. But seriously, just repeating *Anything else?* at intervals? How about a question specific to my case, something to indicate my personal details were registering?

As he started explaining neurofeedback, though, I realized why this wasn't necessary. His technique sounded like a one-size-fits-all procedure. He'd be doing his business the same no matter how I reported my history. Unlike Dr. Pain Specialist, this fellow was kindly and mild-mannered, but I was so tired of struggling to stay nice with people who couldn't seem to help me and were charging me for it too. Doctors should be paying me, I was thinking at this point. I was educational. A fascinating example of *Lingering Brain Damage Due to Prescribed Opioids and Benzodiazepines in a Population of Previously Healthy Individuals.*

I took a deep, shuddering breath and blew it out. "I'm still having trouble with the idea that you guys made me fill out those papers and yet you didn't seem bothered that you were meeting me for the first time without knowing any of my history." They expected me to give 48 hours notice if I couldn't make the appointment; if the packet was so important, why didn't they give me 48 hours notice that it hadn't arrived?

"Yes, we didn't get off to the best start here, did we? But you have to understand—I'm used to people with ADD walking in and

I'll ask about their papers and they'll pull them out of their bag and say, 'Well, I'm *half* done.'"

I regarded him helplessly. "I told your secretary over and over I don't have ADD." Clearly, I was not his usual patient. Once more I was being penalized for following the rules, being the odd one out. "So have you ever had *any* patients like me? People in withdrawal from drugs they took by prescription?"

"Not really," he admitted. He had worked in addiction treatment in the past he said, although that group practice had not employed neurofeedback.

"So how long does it take somebody like me to heal?"

"Well, we used to say that it took two years just to make sure the person stayed off the drugs, and then another three years to repair all the damage they'd done to their lives."

I nodded. I'd heard that sort of thing. But then I shook my head. "That's not me." I looked at Herb. "I haven't messed our lives up too bad yet, have I?"

"No, that's not you."

The doctor pitched his expertise in modest tones, explaining successes he'd had with ADHD children. He repeated two or three times what a steep learning curve there was to the operation of this brain wave regulator. The patient would sit watching a movie, electrodes on her scalp. He would change the picture on the screen in order to make the brain waves adjust to whatever he thought was a more beneficial range or speed. Or something.

"I'm not sure I can buy into this," I said.

"Doesn't matter if you do or not. There's no placebo effect involved. I'm just reprogramming your brain. This was developed by people who figured out how to program landing patterns for airplanes."

I must have grimaced. "It sounds so passive."

"Oh, it is," he said enthusiastically.

"I guess I got all this wrong, then. I thought I was going to be learning to control my own brain waves."

"No, you just sit there watching whatever movie you choose. Patients aren't even aware anything's happening."

I guess this was supposed to be reassuring. No pain. No effort.

But then I realized: "I actually find that frightening—turning my brain over to you."

He smiled and shrugged.

"I mean, my brain's in the messed up shape it's in *because* of all the different drugs I was taking by doctor's prescription."

"But that's the beauty of it, you see. We're not actually putting any drugs in there."

Yeah, got that. But it was this surrendering of control more than the twice-a-week trips here for ten weeks at $100 a pop out of pocket that was giving me qualms.

"Could I maybe just think about this?" I was pretty sure I wouldn't be signing up, but I knew very well I was thinking this on a good day. Next time I was crying in the pit I'd hardly need regret at burning this bridge adding to my misery.

We did not part on the worst of terms. I joked I wasn't sure I could think of enough movies I wanted to watch.

He smiled sheepishly. "Most people like to watch *The Big Bang Theory.*"

Maybe in the end he agreed it wasn't fair to me that he hadn't read or concerned himself with my intake material ahead of my visit.

Likewise, it wouldn't be fair to him to not mention that, without my asking, he later sent me a refund check for the two hundred dollars he'd asked me to pay on my way out his door.

CHAPTER 35

My whole body hummed with optimism that day at the gym. Wednesday, October 15th, 2014. I would mark that date because— hot damn, check it out—I was well! Up to speed with my Group Power class, lifting weights to a Tom Petty cover as I gazed out the huge windows framing the view of my beloved Dimple Hill. Yeah, that's right, like the song said, I'd been stood up at the gates of hell and I hadn't backed down. Shafts of morning light streamed down on the meadow where a doe with twin fawns bounded by. Leaves of the ash trees in the swale had gone golden.

I have a picture of Herb and myself on top of Dimple Hill the autumn before we were married—a selfie the way you had to do it forty years ago, your camera with timer parked in the grass. I framed it inside a little book I made for him, an illustration for the Walt Whitman verse we'd used on our wedding invitations: *Shall we stick by each other as long as we live?*

I added weights to my bar and got ready for the leg strengthening track, thinking how amazingly my life had turned out. It was after Herb and I had each gone off with other people that his one teaching job offer out of forty applications had been in Corvallis. Imagine my surprise when he showed up in Eugene the spring I broke up with my fiancé, explaining that he was teaching middle school in my hometown, occasionally driving by my parents' house, hoping to catch a glimpse of me. Fate, for sure. And this is how, rather than running off to New York City as I had once imagined, I came to be living happily ever after in my own home town.

My God, I loved my husband. I loved my life. There'd never been any component to this long slog through hell that had been about not wanting to be me, blooming right where I'd been planted, with the people I love. The universe was once again smiling on me and, as somebody had been assuring me on one of those CDs of mine, my life was unfolding exactly as it should.

I glanced around at my gym buddies, thrilled to note their names once again popping into my head. Cathy! Eneke! Anne! Oh, how I loved the feeling of a healing brain. I'd thought I was just getting old, but now I could remember things. A sense of new-found power surged through me. Friends had distanced themselves while I'd been sick. So what? I looked around the airy, wood-floored room and smiled at a woman I didn't even know. I'd make new ones.

I jumped in the car and drove home in a kicking-butt-and-taking-names sort of mood, swung up Noley and danced him around. *Who's my pretty baby?* Kid probably thought his grampa had two different wives. Yay! The fun one was back!

That afternoon I told Madeline how we'd finally gotten my mother all moved into her apartment on what was probably the hottest October 6th on record. My brother had stepped up and stayed with her that first night, and she was already loving the apartment and the way the moonlight streamed in her bedroom window at night. Herb had held her hand through closing on her house, so that was that. Mission accomplished.

"Making it to the gym today was my first time ever to get there three times in a row," I told Madeline. "I really think this is it. I'm getting well."

Right.

I would not make it back to the gym for eight months to come.

I cannot recall specifically which symptoms crept up first. The burning nerve pain at the back of my thighs? The realization I was in danger of bursting into tears at some perceived negativity on Herb's part?

I only know that by the next day I'd been smacked back down to the sofa by this cruel message: **You thought you were well but you're not. No matter how good you start to feel, you will always be dragged back. You will lie here sick forever.**

You are doomed.

I watched the TV news that evening as beloved and photogenic nurse Nina Pham was being transported from her Houston hospital and shipped to the National Institutes of Health in Bethesda, Maryland, for treatment of the ebola she had contracted while on duty. Longingly, I regarded the ambulance loading scene—friends and co-workers standing a safe distance on the curb, holding placards bearing slogans of support, affectionately rallying in her time of need.

Then it hit me. Oh, my God—I *envied* her. Given a choice between **frightening, dramatic illness+loving support** and **baffling**

brain damage that scares people away, I'd have switched places with that adorable girl in an instant.

When I was still lying there a week later, watching her get discharged, stopping by the White House for a hug from President Obama, I felt confirmed in my yearnings. A few more weeks and she'd be *Time Magazine's* Person of the Year.

Now it's revealed that the aftermath of ebola is not necessarily uncomplicated, and Nina Pham, suing for damages, claims lingering fatigue, pain, and suffering. I do not envy her this.

I'm admitting to this story only because it shows how bone weary I was of spending so much of my life at the bottom of this pit. Twenty months of post-acute withdrawal syndrome due to withdrawal from Oxycodone and fourteen months since my last Xanax, all things considered, a quick bout of ebola looked good to me.

I spent most of that month on the sofa, flattened by an unrelenting fatigue, the degree of which I had not experienced up to this point. Herb foolishly posited that in spite of my current condition, didn't I really think I was getting better over all?

Good grief.

It was he who had encouraged me the previous spring to reconfigure my detailed health charts, suggesting I pay less attention to tracking every different symptom and simply rate each day **Good, Bad,** or **Mixed.**

"The trend is your friend," he pointed out, borrowing a stock market phrase.

Okay, fine. I would count back any given thirty days, hoping desperately to see some quantifiable improvement. But for six months, every thirty days came out the same—half good days, a quarter bad and a quarter mixed, all of them wildly jerking me upward and plunging me down in a wicked rollercoaster ride that made life difficult to live, impossible to plan.

And now, there it was, plain on my chart. In what world could an uninterrupted thirty-day string of rock-bottom-bad days possibly constitute improvement?

On sleepless, desperate nights I ended up on the sofa where I'd just spent the entire day. I figured Herb didn't need to hear me crying. Better one person on our team got some rest.

After a long, hard cry one time, I fell asleep for the night in the living room and drifted into a toxic nightmare in which I'd been assigned the planning of another wedding for my mother. Once more she would be the bride. The arrangements were about to coalesce, and I reassured her I was heading off to pick up the dress she'd selected.

"Oh, no, I don't want that dress," she said, in the logic of dreams somehow knowing which one I had in mind.

"But it's the one you chose!"

"No, it's not."

My chest gripped in pain. I lowered myself to the stone floor of some unidentifiable cathedral and lay prostrate, cheek against the cold granite, arms spread wide in crucifixion, waiting for the pain to pass, utterly destroyed.

The cold floor morphed into the warm sofa, but that familiar pain jagging up to connect my right jaw with the insufferable clamping of my back and chest wall was real. I struggled to sit up, disentangling myself from the cords of my ever-present heating pad and the buds of my iPod.

I must have been crying out loud, because Herb appeared in the doorframe, backlit.

"How long have you been out here?"

"Um…." I squinted around. "Never made it to bed at all."

"I'm sorry, honey. Guess I conked out before I even noticed."

"It's okay. God. What time is it?"

"Four."

I grimaced. "I've got that scary cramp thing again. And Herb?"

"Yeah?"

I started crying. "I'm so sick of this."

"I know." He helped me up. "C'mon. Let's get you back to bed."

"I can't *do* this anymore."

"Well, you won't have to much longer."

"I mean it. I can't do it one more day."

What could he say? He'd already heard this hundreds of times, would hear it hundreds more.

He tucked me back in under the covers, climbed in on his side and wrapped his arms around me. "Is it going away?"

"Yeah, it's better."

"It didn't last very long, right?"

"Huh uh," I murmured, feeling safe again, drifting off directly into another dream.

The many long lines at the Department of Motor Vehicles dismayed me. Which queue to join? Apparently I was here to renew my driver's license, but everyone I begged for directions looked right past me. I felt not so much invisible as that I had been deemed by the crowd as completely unworthy of attention. Shuffling forward, I finally reached some official-looking person who demanded my current license. I opened my wallet. Oh, no! It wasn't there! I was impatiently ordered aside, where I stood at a chest-high counter, frantically going through my wallet, which, like a circus car spilling clowns, was comically producing more than it ever could have held. Dozens of clipped images from vintage greeting cards, a picture of me in slimmer, prettier days. But not the license. Not my official identification. Not the thing I needed to prove I was a person who should be entitled to drive, to move forward, to live again. I could not find myself.

But, wait. What the—? Suddenly I was holding a complicated new cell phone, the type I'd been tentatively promising I'd learn to use. Maybe Herb bought it, so quick as he always was to research and put in hand anything that might help me. Okay, so I'd call him. Maybe he'd have an idea where I might have left my photo ID. I tapped in some numbers. No, wrong. Try again. Still wrong. Try again. Okay, got it. But, *shit*. Now I couldn't find the send button. Oh, give it up. What a hopeless loser.

And then the truly scary implication of this hit me. No ID meant I'd have to drive home without my license. That was illegal! I would be in big trouble!

Panicked, I burst into tears. Right there in the DMV I was melting down, sinking to the floor with my fingers clutching the edge of the counter. I just couldn't do this. I couldn't do it anymore....

I woke up sobbing. The fact that Herb's arms were still wrapped around me meant I probably hadn't been asleep any time at all.

During this stretch I made it to town only three times—twice for acupuncture and once to talk to Madeline. Herb hauled me over to the kids' house for a pumpkin carving party, but it did nothing to perk me up, and I'm sure I wasn't much fun.

Day after day I lay on the sofa, not sleeping, yet too exhausted to do anything. Was that me who last summer on my good days scraped a decade's worth of moss off the brick patio? Cleaned and repainted the garden gates and the wooden wagon wheel leaning against the picket fence? Put in a couple of days hacking the invasive English ivy out of Mary's and Jaci's new backyard in Portland? Finally succeeded in shoveling out Herb's pack-rat office and turning it into a lovely room for the baby?

Totally deluded not to see and accept it: I was not getting better, I was getting worse.

This is when one of the most persistent fears of people in withdrawal from benzodiazepines hit me hardest. Good God, I must have something else. The dread of chronic fatigue came tingling up the back of my legs, snaked into my brain and hissed dark poison.

But no, I wasn't about to go back to any of my old doctors or look for a new one. I couldn't bear the thought of re-telling my long and tortuous story one more time to somebody trying to fit me into a set of boxes and a fifteen minute time slot. I was even more weary of trying to explain it to well-meaning friends who might casually question whether I had really tried hard enough to find the *right* doctor.

Time had never passed more slowly. This was worse than when I'd been put to bed with high blood pressure seven weeks prior to Miles's birth. I couldn't sleep, I could only lie there, sinking deeper and deeper into this dark hole, this traumatizing silence, every moment feeling less connected to the world. My brain had done fight or flight mode; now it was closing in, shutting down.

All the muscles of my back ached. It felt like some live and menacing thing was actually clinging to me. Was this, I wondered dimly, where the expression "monkey on my back" came from?

Physical pain, however, was nothing compared to trying to endure the utterly bleak state of my mind. Even with Herb in the next room, I felt completely alone. I thought of all those suffering souls kept captive in solitary confinement. I was one with them. Once, I remember feeling I was just as close to being in a coma as was possible without it being official. I wasn't moving, hardly breathing. What if I just quietly slipped over that line? Could I? Maybe being in an actual coma wouldn't be the worst thing. They'd have to rush me to the hospital, set me up where I could be carefully guarded. The people who in the past had claimed to love me might come around and hold my hands and urge me to hang on. They'd say the words I needed to hear to contradict the sick voices in my head. I'd tried, but I couldn't seem to get my family to understand how desperately I craved a listing of some specific reasons why I, in particular, was a human being worth keeping alive.

If I ever knew these things for myself, over and over, down in the dark, I felt perilously close to forgetting forever.

CHAPTER 36

The BenzoBuddies site had been created in 2004 by a benzo survivor from Yorkshire, England, a very private man who wanted to help others. And help he did. Many credit this community of strangers with saving their lives.

I'd been randomly scanning its posts for a year-and-a-half, often in the middle of the night, taking comfort in the confirmation that the symptoms I was experiencing were not uncommon in benzo withdrawal. I never signed on to request support or tell my own story; I just accepted for myself the encouragement written for others. I'd eventually read enough, after all, to have a pretty good handle on what those words would be if I asked for them.

One day in November, though, I came across a frantic post from someone who described what sounded like the very sort of chest cramping anxiety episodes I'd been experiencing. It seemed wrong to withhold the reassurance that I could give, the confirmation that mine were diminishing in frequency and intensity. So, in order to post, I finally joined.

What an eye-opening business, making my membership official. Now, with everyone's avatars and drug history "signatures" popping up, the ghostlike, commiserating internet voices became real people, individuals coming through sharp and plaintive, desperate with the appalling details of consignment to hell by way of their doctor's prescriptions.

Here were my fellow prisoners, each locked in a cell under solitary confinement. In a high-rise overlooking the bay in Halifax, Nova Scotia, a garden within hearing of the foghorns on San Francisco Bay. From the wealthiest zip code in Connecticut to the much reduced circumstances of somebody's faulty-furnaced trailer in rural Ohio. From Norway, where the long hours of winter darkness would seem to invite depression, to Florida and Laguna Beach, California, where the sunshine wasn't cheering up a couple of guys in benzo withdrawal the slightest bit. Scotland, Ireland, England, New Zealand, Chile, Italy, Spain, France, Austria, Germany, Mexico, New York City, Toronto, Michigan, Hawaii, Oklahoma City, Vancouver, B.C.....one guy straight down Territorial Highway from me, right here in Oregon.

Each person seemed to be their doctor's sole patient who'd had such difficulties in withdrawal from benzodiazepines. Most were told what they were going through in trying to get off of the drugs couldn't possibly be related to the drugs themselves. Often, additional psych drugs would be added or the dose of the original drug increased.

It takes a lot of guts to stand up to a figure of authority condescendingly implying that, sadly, *you* are the mentally ill person in this exam room, while *he* is the highly-educated keeper of knowledge. It's especially hard to be brave when you're already feeling sick and beaten down. People tentatively explaining to their doctors about finding on-line support and advice for safely tapering off their drugs were invariably warned to steer clear of the internet, that people on forums such as BenzoBuddies all had pre-existing mental health issues not related to benzos.

Not true! *I* was on BenzoBuddies. My friend Lynne, perfectly sane and solid, mother and grandmother, deacon in our church, had found her best help from strangers here when she suffered from Klonopin withdrawal. Of course there were people with long, tangled drug histories, some involving abuse, but the vast majority of people had arrived at this juncture simply by following their doctors' orders, many accepting a benzo prescription in hopes of sleeping a bit better, or to calm anxiety about getting on a plane for an important trip. These were smart, literate, creative people. Or had been before benzos compromised their brains. Teachers, nurses, writers, lawyers, scientists, business entrepreneurs and executives, therapists, spacecraft technologists, real estate agents, college students, actors and musicians.

The stories that most outraged me were those of people who'd been started on these drugs for some off-label use like restless leg syndrome or tinnitus who, when they became suicidal in withdrawal, were told that this was merely their underlying anxiety now coming to the forefront. Never mind that they'd never had a desperate mental moment in their lives until they fell into the pit of Big Pharma.

Perhaps the most poignant were women who'd been put on benzos to help them cope with chemotherapy. Now they had survived, but claimed that nothing in their cancer treatments came anywhere close to the horrors of benzo withdrawal. It was heartbreaking too, to read of young mothers trying to care for new babies while so critically compromised, or women who, out of necessity, were having to launch into withdrawal because of a pregnancy.

The men on the board had their own masculine slant on despair. They felt themselves up against a powerful opponent, and *brutal* was a word frequently used to describe the physical and mental pain of withdrawal. It was especially difficult for the young men, formerly strong and athletic, who were outraged at the idea of being *brought to their knees* (another oft-used phrase) by a tiny pill. I felt for them. I'm sure being bedridden with an illness the outside world views with skepticism does not feel one bit manly.

Yes, "thinking of others" is supposed to be beneficial for a person, actually increasing the production of dopamine, serotonin, oxcytocin—the good stuff. My mother had always taught me never to miss the chance to pass on a compliment, reach out and send a note if you heard someone had hit a rocky patch. And by all means, acknowledge everyone's birthday in a timely fashion. But in withdrawal, my tenuous grip on myself had often made it impossible for me to get any further down my own list than the one item right there at the top: **Live through this day.** Or sometimes: **Live through this hour.**

But now, here were people going through exactly what I had been, their stories validating the difficulty of this strange struggle. Whether they had family surrounding them or were trying to get through this entirely on their own, one thing everyone had in common was this: nobody felt understood. Even people with ostensibly the best possible support systems felt that only the people on the BenzoBuddies board really got it, the horror of their moment-to-moment mental suffering, why it was so impossible for them to simply cheer up and be their old selves, as their families repeatedly, earnestly recommended they should. It was touching how people took pains to answer with encouragement the people who posted in terrible distress. Especially appreciated were the ones who returned to write success stories, explaining how sick they'd been, how much they were enjoying their lives now that they'd healed.

Reading the long, tortuous routes by which people had finally come to understand that no, they did not have chronic fatigue syndrome, no, they did not have fibromyalgia, no, they did not have MS, but that prescribed meds were at the root of their problems, I realized I had actually been *lucky* in having had enough trouble with opioid withdrawal that it had occurred to me to explore whether I had inadvertently become addicted to benzos as well. I could so easily have been one of those people just continuing to keep Xanax in what I thought of as my little Toolkit for Dealing with Life, unaware I was teaching my brain to be incapable of putting me to sleep without it, never associating certain symptoms with benzo tolerance.

People would write of their distress over a particularly cruel withdrawal symptom known as "intrusive thoughts." Naturally no one wanted to upset others with graphic depictions of their own personal horror scenarios, so this remained hypothetical for me. But one day a post from one of the moderators gave a definition of intrusive thoughts, mentioning they might be flashing images of self harm.

Okay, this was late in the game for me to put it all together, but I instantly thought of three separate instances, the year *before* my surgery, where I'd experienced this, no doubt while in tolerance to Xanax.

Once, in the fall, we'd parked our car on the roof of a parking structure at PDX on our way to visit Aunt Catherine in Los Angeles. I do not remember the specific life circumstances to which I was ascribing my immediate gloom; I remember only looking across the pavement at the lot's three-foot cement barricade at the edge and flashing on the notion that dashing over and vaulting it might not be the worst idea in the world.

Reporting this to Herb only annoyed him, so, inside the terminal, I put in a call to Mary, and begged her to remind me that she would not take kindly to any such drastic measures on my part.

Shortly after that I'd insisted on having my thyroid checked again, and found I was once more out of whack. When an adjustment in my dosage brought prompt relief, it was easy enough to attribute this weird episode entirely to my thyroid.

The next spring, however, it happened again. While cleaning up the old homestead site at Kitten Creek, I looked at a scattering of glass in the mud and flashed on the idea of snatching up a shard and raking it across my wrist. I never so much as bent and reached for it, but the thought itself seemed completely bizarre. My healthy brain would never be thinking anything but how best to get on with the business of cleaning up the garbage.

So what did I do to calm myself down? Took a Xanax, of course! It worked quickly, perfectly, telling me, *See? This is all in your head. Just some sort of anxiety thing.*

It never occurred to me this was Xanax itself saying, *Good girl, you knew you'd gone too long without taking me. Don't let it be so long again.*

The third time I was under my favorite ancient Doug fir. I had my pruning saw, and as I looked up at a dangling branch—a widow-maker—the risky stupidity of standing there without my hard hat crossed my mind.

Ah, but, on the other hand, wouldn't it just be easier if that branch dropped right on my head and put me out of my misery?

Breep breep! Wrong thought, wrong thought.

Upset, I told Herb.

His response?

"Well, I've got your hard hat right there in the truck."

I'll never forget that, and *I've got your hardhat right there in truck* has become my private code for *Wow, you are not getting what I'm trying to say at all, are you?*

Another time that spring, Herb and I had gone to Portland and had lunch with some friends at a nice downtown restaurant. Afterwards, walking back to our car, I was suddenly taken ill. Reluctant to give up on the rest of the afternoon's errands, we proceeded to Filson's for woods-working clothes. But why wasn't Herb hanging onto me in the parking strip? Couldn't he see I was dizzy and close to dropping in my tracks? I ended up too sick and scared to shop. We next tried heading across the Hawthorne Bridge to visit Herb's favorite bookstore, Murder by the Book, soon to close. I hated to rob Herb—surely one of the store's best customers—of a last chance to walk out with a big grocery sack full of mysteries.

But I couldn't hack it. "I'm sorry, honey, I'm too sick."

"You wanna just go home?"

I nodded, shutting my eyes. Was I having a heart attack? Certainly something was going on. Traffic stalled while we were trying to get back over the bridge. Maybe I was dying. Maybe I needed to go to an emergency room. I rolled my head and looked at Herb with half-closed eyes.

"Pretty bad?"

I nodded.

"You better tell me what to do," he said.

Oh, my God. What if I passed out? Would he be shaking me, begging for a decision? Was this guy I married capable of getting me to a hospital if I were dying but couldn't say so?

Finally the traffic began to move and we got back on I-5.

"Can you pull over?" I managed.

"Right now?"

Jesus. "Uh, when it's safe?"

At some suburban exit he parked next to a curb edging a green lawn. I opened the door, leaned out and vomited.

So, food poisoning. What else could it be? And yet when we checked later, no one else at the lunch was ill, even my friend Tami, who'd eaten the exact salad I'd had. And didn't food poisoning take longer to develop?

It seems so clear now: this was a classic panic attack. But how was I to know? I'd never had any such thing in my life. The possibility never occurred to me until I went on the BenzoBuddies Forum and read stories of all the misdiagnosed illnesses people suffered from in the grip of benzo tolerance and withdrawal.

It was not long after that, when my knee blew out with the inevitable arthritis after all my previous surgeries and I felt the PTSD of that whole chronic pain/depression/repeated-surgeries episode barking at my heels, that I caved and asked to go on the antidepressant Lexapro. My brain was not right. And I was not ignorant. I knew I should not be thinking these life-loathing thoughts, and if it was still happening with my thyroid in check, then maybe my doctors were right that I should be on antidepressants.

Now, unraveling my own history, it seems clear to me that the antidepressant, combined with the benzo, conspired to keep the opioids from giving me the needed pain relief after my knee-replacement surgery, thus making it necessary to take such a high dose of Oxycodone for so long.

So it all went back to the Xanax.

But now I had it figured it out. My brain was clean. When it finally healed from the after effects, I would be well.

Let's pause for a moment here to pity any doctor in my future who unwittingly suggests prescribing me or anybody I love a benzo, and then tries to claim it's perfectly safe.

CHAPTER 37

＞———————————＜

Experienced writing teachers sometimes encourage neophytes by explaining it's not necessary to have the course of an entire book in mind before starting to write. One may drive a long journey in the dark, they point out, seeing only as far ahead at any given time as the headlights cast their beams.

Nice metaphor for the writing of a novel, but it certainly didn't fit for my dreary situation. The distance of headlight beams? Ha! I felt like I was trying to live my life with a scrim hung a mere foot in front of my face, as if I were not allowed to envision anything at all beyond the present horrid moment.

But at last I remember a certain day, lying on the sofa, still wasted with fatigue, when I nevertheless noticed something new and interesting going on in my brain. What was that warm little buzzing? Could it be—? Wow, I was actually thinking about the future, a future where I was miraculously well. I probably still looked like a half-dead person—not that anyone was watching—but somewhere in there a little spark had flared up. I was making plans, plotting projects I would do, dance classes I would attend, books I would write.

Optimism, that's what it's called, and you can't feel it without dopamine. Maybe those neurotransmitters were producing some again. Maybe my brain was staging a comeback!

Until my body agreed to go along, though, I couldn't even begin to put any of those plans into action.

Will decided to go house hunting in Bend, and I had to content myself with being allowed to run real estate searches on-line and forward him the listings. I had to limit myself to studying Google street photos when what I really wanted to do was jump in the car, drive over the pass and check out those houses with him myself. Not that he needed me for this. He found the perfect place on his own. But it would it would have been fun.

When would I ever be a person capable of fun again? I was still so sick, so fatigued. I couldn't go anywhere. My Visa bill was the statement of a dead woman. No lunches. No project supplies—no paint, no wallpaper. No clothes ordered with optimistic visions of outings and occasions in the future. When it registered on the computers at Sundance, Anthropologie and Johnny Was that I'd stopped perusing their sites and making impulse purchases, they plaintively messaged me—*We miss you!* Yeah, I missed me too.

All those long, winter weeks I lay tethered to my heating pad in the living room. But call it the not-living room. The wasting-away room. I probably looked like a grayed-out "before" in a TV commercial for antidepressants, a sad and aging person painfully aware that life was going by somewhere beyond the confines of my house.

It helped to learn from BenzoBudies that my drastic turn for the worse at this point was not at all unusual. Much discussion was devoted to the completely baffling non-linear nature of the brain's healing. A common post of despair would come from someone who'd been feeling so well, they thought they were healed, only to find themselves, as I had, thrown back into the pit.

And the fresh array of new symptoms I was experiencing at seventeen months off Xanax was apparently not unusual either. I had weird inner vibrations, attacks of racing heartbeat, itchy rashes, another round of stomach trouble, weird and striking shoulder pains when I'd never had issues with my shoulders in my life. A symptom I found particularly distressing was the overall body stiffness. I felt like I was a hundred years old. Was this just what aging felt like and I was a deluded idiot, hoping to ever dance again?

Each day some crude, diabolical chef plated these ever-rotating combinations of symptoms for me saying, *This is it for today. Eat it. You wanna side of adrenal aches with that? Ya save room for heart palps?*

Sometimes it felt like I had two parallel pipes running under my skin from my shoulders down my backside to my heels into which liquid pain would periodically be poured, there to burn. When the time for that prescribed torture ended, valves at my heels would open for the pain to swiftly drain away.

Mostly I slept well, but several times, after a string of decent days, I'd be awakened in the middle of the night as if the withdrawal truck had once more run me over, brutally delivering the news that no, despite my best hopes, I was not yet well.

One night I dreamed Herb had dropped me off at the church for some kind of ladies' social. I ran into Lynne, my real-life BB friend, and as I was updating her on my current health status, a woman from another cluster of people overheard me.

"I know exactly what you need to do," she said.

I turned expectantly, eager to hear some bit of magically healing advice. The woman was quite thin, wearing—weirdly of course—a pale green leotard and tights.

"What you need to do," she said, "is just start really *trying*."

Trying? *Trying?*

Enraged, I grabbed her. I flung her toothpick body to the floor and, sobbing, started pummeling and choking her. On one hand, I was thinking I didn't even know how to beat up a person. On the other, if I didn't get a grip, I could have pounded her to death. Apparently my better nature prevailed, because I released her and she scrambled up. Crouching away, keeping a wary eye on me, she started whispering about me to the rest of the guests, just in case they hadn't seen this shocking bit of drama.

Then Herb showed up all sweet and hopeful.

"Did you have fun, Honey?"

I tilted my forehead against his chest in shame and confessed I had pretty much torn it with the whole town now, because I had publicly taken down the hostess. I had beat up a woman in church.

CHAPTER 38

————————————

"Help!"

So strange to find myself finally yelling aloud what had been running as a humming plea through my head for over two years by now. *Would somebody for God's sake please help me?*

And now the Fed-Ex man was just going to turn his back, get in his truck and drive away?

I balanced on what had since one hour ago become my better leg.

"Help!"

But he didn't get in the truck. He was only slamming the door. He turned toward me, took steps in my direction.

"Linda? Is that you out there?"

Oh, thank God. He was coming. And it was the guy who knew me, Mike, the one who was always so nice and told me his wife liked my books.

I burst into tears of relief, which he apparently read as pain.

"No, no, I'm okay. It's just that this is so stupid." I was crying for the utter absurdity of managing to injure myself just when it seemed like maybe I was finally getting well.

"Okay, stay put," he said. "I'll back the truck up to the greenhouse so you'll only have to go a few more steps."

I watched Mike maneuver the truck as close as possible.

Dammit. I'd been trying, right? On any day I wasn't smacked with fatigue or pain I'd been trying to psych myself out, pretend to be a well person. Just go out there and hack around in the trees like I normally would…..

Mike came and had me put my right arm over his shoulder.

"It's too bad it wasn't Jason Summers doing this route today," he said apologetically. "He's six-two, works out all the time. He could have picked you right up."

"Yeah?" I was laughing and crying at the same time. "Sounds kinda thrilling, but you know what? Since my husband can't carry me, it's probably just as well you can't either."

Note to self: If you're thinking of having any more accidents where you need to be carried, try to ditch some weight and not be such a pudgy little challenge.

In his truck, Mike ferried me across the road and up the drive to our front porch, then helped me up the brick steps, where I lowered myself to the bench, injured ankle outstretched. This sweet guy waited with me until Herb showed up a few minutes later. Where were the cameras? Could have made a nice PR ad for Fed-Ex.

We spent the afternoon at Immediate Care, me alternately weeping and laughing at the absurdity of this. A sweet Chinese-American nurse took down the details of my accident.

"Did you hit your head?" she asked, her tone grave.

"No," I said, understanding now why this was so important. Without your brain, you've got nothing.

When the designated doctor popped her head in the door we saw it was Robin Lannan, who'd been in a ninth-grade English class Herb taught when he was twenty-four.

"We all had such a crush on you," she told him.

Well, of course they did. As we waited for x-rays, Herb reminded me she'd been part of a group of the smartest girls at Cheldelin Middle School. They knew perfectly well who was crush-worthy!

By the time we were back in her office awaiting the results, Herb and I had agreed my injury was probably just a sprain. Then Dr. Lannan pushed open the door.

"I'm sorry, but you've broken your ankle."

I started crying again. As if Herb and I could have agreed what the outcome on this should be and that's how it would go. The only bright spot I could see was that I hadn't broken it stepping into the rodent holes of Herb's gated garden as I'd warned him I surely would. Kindly placating me, he had finally rototilled that ground to a safer smoothness. Clever me, managing to find another way to get the ankle-breaking job done—a molehill, it would turn out.

I don't know what it said in my medical records regarding narcotic painkillers, but despite everybody apparently assuming my tears were about pain and not epic frustration, nobody asked me if I wanted a prescription for opioids.

Fine. I didn't.

I was pretty miserable that night. It took a lot of hard crying to express the rage I felt at what seemed to me such a sharp arrow of outrageous fortune. I thought I'd been just about ready to ramp up the exercise regime that would speed my healing process. Now I faced six weeks of holding perfectly still, burning about five calories per hour.

In the middle of the night, though, I woke up with something amazing going on. The words of this book were again pouring into my head. I had to get going and write them down.

In the morning, I told Herb my plan. My brain felt healed and that's all I needed to finish my book. A broken ankle wouldn't hold me back. In fact, didn't this give me a pass from pitching in with any and all housework? Something I would have killed for as a young mother, trying to carve out time to write? I would never insist to anyone including myself that everything happens for a reason, but I do believe in making the best of whatever *does* come along. So now I could pretend I had been accepted to a lovely writer's retreat, the kind where they leave a basket of sandwiches on your cottage steps for lunch. I'd always wished for that. Now it was simply being delivered in a slightly altered form, a couple of decades later.

Herb didn't miss a beat. He got Miles to come over and help fashion a temporary office at the end of the long, narrow living room. They carried my computer equipment down from my upstairs office and put it on my little oak drop-leaf desk, the one I'd bought at an auction when we were first married to use for my writing. He put my printer on the heirloom children's table where I used to park Mary and Willie for lunch. Lamps, wastebasket, the little Mr. Coffee one-cup hot plate Will had given me for Christmas years ago—Herb thought of everything.

I can hardly express how much this support meant to me. He was confirming my intentions, agreeing that I probably had something worthwhile to say that ought to be written down. That I still had a mind worthy of encouragement.

Having a broken ankle was amazingly eye-opening. Everyone was so swift to be kind. I saw it before we even left the clinic the day of the accident. Sit in a wheelchair with your leg propped up and watch the sympathy automatically flow right your way.

On Sunday morning Mike, the Fed-Ex man, stopped by with an elegant little potted orchid, wanting to check on my outcome. So glad to give him such a definitive report! Yes, my ankle was officially broken! He wouldn't have to backpedal on the story he'd told his wife.

In the days ahead, more flowers appeared. I received cards and sick visits. Mary drove down from Portland with fingerless mittens she'd knitted—perfect for popping on the bare toes peeking out from my cast. Who knew a broken bone was such a popular predicament? I'd been so sick, for so long, but now I'd managed to mangle myself in such a way as to punch the proper *pay attention* buttons in people. Call the florist! Hit the Hallmark store! I took comfort in this confirmation that I was still a person who qualified for demonstrations of care and concern as long as I had the good grace to present with a fully comprehensible malady, an injury that apparently happened to many perfectly nice people.

As Dr. Kliewer told me so long ago, we live on hope.

People always insist they're protecting themselves from disappointment by carefully refusing to get their hopes up. I say, to hell with that. Get your hopes up. Early and often. If things don't go the way you secretly want, you'll be bummed whether you've admitted your hopes to yourself or not. And once you figure out there's no

Tribunal of the Universe waiting to punish you for having the audacity to root for yourself and say so, why not?

Now it was time for me to practice the philosophy I had given my own heroine, Lovisa King, in my Oregon Trail novel, *A Heart for Any Fate*—that the best way to come out of something as a survivor is to do your best to *act* like somebody who's hanging tight to the faith that you will. I buckled down to writing my book, teasing myself along with the story of how fate would undoubtedly allow my final withdrawal symptoms to dissipate just about the time I got my cast off.

Didn't happen. Not even close.

For starters, a broken ankle in a period of feeling good, a window, was a mere riffle in the river carrying my little boat along. When the next wave of symptoms hit, a broken ankle on top of withdrawal felt like I'd gone straight over a waterfall and smashed onto the rocks below. I lay there, immobilized in every possible way. My poor brain hardly knew which part to work on healing first.

And the reality that I didn't know then—thanks again for not being able to see the future—was that my ankle would be healed and ancient history long before I finally rounded the last bend that would put opioid and benzo brain damage behind me and out of sight for good.

During this time though, down deep, the healing was happening, and once in awhile I'd be tossed a little life-ring of hope.

Eighteen months to the day since I quit taking Xanax, I hobbled to the living room to write. As the morning sun streamed in through the lace-curtained window by the piano and struck the oak desk of my makeshift office, I was visited by a lovely thought. For several days I had awakened with my native optimism in full force, my mind glowing with a precious kernel of power and confidence. I knew this feeling, but I hadn't felt it with quite this intensity since I was newly pregnant with Miles, walking around town, this amazing, invisible secret within me. As if I were the first woman ever to have conceived.

Now I felt that same way.

I had a secret. I had conceived.

I was luminously pregnant with my own long-sought rebirth.

I thought wellness would announce itself with ever-longer strings of good days. Instead, in May, it sneaked up on me with the absence of bad ones. I had stopped falling into the pit, and if I wasn't going to be slammed down and crying every few days, maybe I could see about getting some traction on living my life again.

I had the windows washed. I called in a service to clean the bedroom carpet in the room where I had spent far too many hours, curled on the brass bed, crying. I had the living room sofa cleaned too. I'm not sure it was even dirty. I didn't care. I'd spent all those endless hours there with my heating pad and a DVD player, and I wanted a symbolic end to that. I wanted a fresh start.

I even took the Subaru in for detailing. With green Oregon moss growing over the back window, I'll bet it was the dirtiest car they'd ever cleaned.

When I went into the office to pay, the manager asked how my day was going.

"Excellent." I was beaming. "Just excellent."

"Really. Wow, I don't usually hear that."

Yeah, well, he probably wasn't usually dealing with people who'd been down in the dark so long that going out and claiming a clean car could be regarded as an experience of such astonishing delight.

On Friday, June 5th, I popped a Jake Shimabukuro CD into the player of my spiffy clean Subaru and headed across town to reactivate my Timberhill Athletic Club membership. I hadn't played this CD of catchy ukulele music in ages. It sounded…triumphant! It sounded the way I felt.

When I got home I wrote and posted my "success" story on the BenzoBuddies board.

A couple of days later, we climbed in the loaded pick-up truck at first light and headed for the cabin. I had an important job—the clearing of a path to the creek for a certain beloved little family member of ours.

When I walked into the cabin, I laughed as I always do, delighted anew with all my treasured Oregon Trail décor. But this time it truly hit me. This whole project had somehow come together in the three years I'd been sick. It was as if somebody pretending to be me had been here and fixed everything up, just the way she knew I'd like it.

I went out onto the porch, took one long look at the western ridge-top horizon, and burst into tears.

Relief. I had survived.

CHAPTER 39

People shouldn't have to go through this.

Not opioid withdrawal.

Not benzo withdrawal.

Not when those first pills come by way of a doctor's prescription pad.

Not when those drugs were urged upon these doctors by friendly and attractive young pharmaceutical representatives who are delighted to pay for lunch, but who can provide no studies of long term outcomes for all the unsuspecting and doomed patients; reps who, indeed, are coached to minimize the suspected side effects of the drugs they're pushing.

I would love to join a class action lawsuit against a few pharmaceutical companies. Isn't this where the true cynicism festers, in the deliberate obscuring of scientific evidence in favor of profit? We could start with Purdue Pharma, the makers of Oxycodone, whose reps assured doctors their amazing new painkiller would addict less than one per cent of their patients.

And shouldn't somebody go in and do some kick-butt housekeeping at the FDA? Follow the money. Allowing federal officials tasked with approving new drugs to nurture financial ties to the pharmaceutical industry itself is a perfectly lousy prescription. It's not one bit nice to turn the constituency you're charged with protecting into a miserable bunch of lab rats.

Everyone's different. How many times had I heard that? But whether cursed by a predisposition to immediately crave more of any given dopamine producing substance or not, none can consider themselves proof against the power of narcotics. Take a potent opioid painkiller for any length of time at all and your brain will rebel without it. Whether you know why you feel so miserable, or simply fret you've had the bad luck to contract the flu first thing out of the hospital post-surgery, the fact is, you are suffering from withdrawal.

Baby boomers will be undergoing joint replacement surgeries in ever greater numbers in the coming years, and I wouldn't want my story to scare anyone away from doing this. I like my new knee; I just wish I hadn't had to spend three-and-a-half years recovering from pharmaceuticals to get to the point where I could be appreciating it. Surely most patients will not need the high doses of painkillers I did in order to overcome the blocking properties of the antidepressant and the benzo I was on. And I hope doctors will awaken to the realization that true kindness to their patients is to stand firm against the casual refilling of prescriptions for pain relief, even if at the conclusion of that post-op visit, it seems like the friendliest, most expedient way to usher us out the door.

A study by the pharmacy benefits manager Express Scripts reported in the New York Times December 9, 2014, found that nearly half the people who took painkillers for whatever reason for a minimum of thirty days were still taking them *three years later.* Now that's an addictive substance.

Even without the issues I encountered, plenty of people having knee-replacement surgery are going to be on narcotics for that thirty days or more. Crunch the numbers and you come up with some alarming statistics on the number of people potentially becoming addicted.

On October 22, 2013, the very day I was, myself, sitting in the office of the doctor specializing in addiction, a man about my age posted to the internet a summation of his recent experience with knee replacement surgery. Overall he was pleased with his new knees and looked forward to resuming his active lifestyle. But his concluding statement jumped out at me:

The worst part of this whole thing was withdrawal from Oxycodone. I really wish I had been counseled by my doctor about this drug and just what it can do to you.

Exactly. Could we please address the issue of informed consent? Doctors, you need to be explaining to patients the potential side effects of these drugs. Stop couching the debate as simply one of deciding which patients are "nice enough" to be trusted with these prescriptions. Stop consoling yourselves with the pharmaceutical industry's reassurance that you have not turned a healthy person into a drug addict, you have merely rendered her "physically dependent."

Physical dependence on opioids is not a benign condition. It is not, as you have been encouraged to believe, clinically insignificant. Know this: the patient you so cavalierly dismiss from your office with this diagnosis may very well be facing the most difficult challenge of her life.

In contrast to opioids, an individual's reaction to benzos and the difficulty of withdrawing from them seems to vary more widely across the population, but judging from the level of suffering of those with the bad genetic luck to have horrific reactions to short term use and long, drawn-out timelines for healing after discontinuation, it seems criminal that twenty years after protocols for prescribing these drugs began to advise limiting use to two to four weeks, doctors in the United States are still writing open-ended prescriptions and casually approving refills.

Doctors, please resist the temptation to be the savior who brings sleep to insomniacs by way of Xanax or a similar benzo. An Australian doctor, proud of never initiating such a prescription, suggests that anyone considering doing so should explain it to their patients like this: *Yes, I can give you something which will help you sleep. It works very well. The only catch is, I'll be turning you into a drug addict.*

And if the patient tries to free herself of the drug, who knows how far her mind will career away from her? I'd like to suggest that a doctor should never prescribe a drug without articulating a timeline of expected use, an understanding of what it takes to get *off* of that drug, and a willingness to help the patient accomplish this. No fair claiming, as some doctors reportedly have, that they assumed the patient understood going on a certain benzo meant being on it for life. Seriously? Get it in writing.

What if the only difference between physical dependence and addiction is that in physical dependence, the doctor has had the personal good luck to addict a patient who will suffer quietly through a miserable recovery without giving him any trouble or ever calling him to account?

I was, after all, the Good Girl who didn't raid anybody's medicine cabinet.

And Good Girls are nice, as everyone knows. They sit down and shut up.

Yeah? Can't make me. Something about having to haul myself through this without the aid of any authorities also healed me from my lifelong fear of them.

I never thought of suing on my own. No amount of money could ever give me back the time I've lost or serve as reparations for my mental distress. It has always meant more to me to tell this story, which, as everyone who's survived it will attest, can be nothing short of a harrowing existential crisis, the fight of our lives.

You won't be surprised at my dismay to discover that even many consecutive days of euphoric wellness do not, in benzo recovery, guarantee against the reappearance of symptoms. Over and over in the course of the next year I would again find myself bursting into happy tears, with that sense of finally having come home from a long, perilous journey. But, as every screenwriter knows, tears of joy come only when the outcome up to that very instant has been gravely in doubt, so for every time I looked at Herb across the dinner table and burst into tears of relief, it was only because, briefly at least, the happy outcome had once more seemed less than certain.

But at least I finally learned to stop being appalled. None of this could shock me anymore. I embraced what some refer to as radical acceptance.

I took care of myself. I made a healing ritual of doing yoga every morning in an upstairs, light-flooded room, always accompanied by the same soothing soundtrack—*Music to Inspire Positive*

Thinking. During floor poses on a sun-warmed patch of the rose-patterned Persian carpet, I took in the sky show out the double windows: scudding clouds, wind lashing the trees, morning sun slanting through at ever-changing angles. In upward dog I could watch a squirrel bouncing on the bare branch of the walnut tree, a V of geese, a hawk settling on the pinnacle of the tallest Doug fir. When I stood up for warrior, I could look down and see my little grandson outside, digging in the daffodils. The crabapple arching over the patio did its brief but sweetly perfect blooming right outside the left window pane.

I read books on my Kindle about the benefits of exercise while I pedaled the stationary bike. If something upset me and made my blood pressure spike, I jumped on my mini-trampoline for an episode of *How I Met Your Mother* (second time through) or ordered myself out to do a loop of the trees at a fast clip. Worked like charm. At the crack of dawn I did a trampoline stint in the backyard to Jesse Colin Young's joyous "Morning Sun" (helped me feel 23 again!) and Carly Simon's triumphant "Let the River Run."

I became an excellent boss of myself. I wasn't bad as the compliant patient, either.

I worked in the woods when I could, found something useful to do requiring less physical energy when I couldn't. If all bets were off—something which happened with less frequency as the months passed—I lay down with my heating pad on the sofa and watched the latest from Netflix. No harm, no foul.

I no longer needed to listen to *Meditations on Anger and Forgiveness* quite so often. In my darkest hours I'd truly feared the ability to forgive would be forever beyond me, but it turned out that forgiveness for simple cluelessness on the part of those who should have known better came easily once the horror of forever feeling ill was replaced by the sweet peace of recovery.

I read books about healing the brain. I tried to feed mine only images of beauty and stories of hope. I arranged my space so that everywhere I looked my eye would fall upon some token of my loved ones, those who I now did feel were rooting for me.

In spite of my earlier claims concerning the superiority of female empathy, I ended up receiving some of the most reliable support from the men in my family. They had long ago accepted the general cultural condemnation that as men, they couldn't hope to understand women, but when it became apparent that I was expecting from them not some formulation of magic words that would instantly cure me, but rather was hoping simply for the steady of reassurance of their caring and concern, they all came through.

I cherished the new tenderness in Miles's demeanor. I'd always figured he'd never quite understand how we'd felt about him until he had that firstborn child of his own. Now he got it. And he lost at least a bit of his taste for arguing with me. After all, we agreed on the most important thing, that he'd been right in his prediction: Nolan was the most awesome baby ever.

I doubt Herb's brother John realized how much his sympathetic emails on the general theme of *I'm rooting for you* meant to me. Like his big brother, he'd instinctively stumbled on what I most needed to hear.

As for Will—ever since a birthday visit when I'd confessed my desperation, how much I needed my family hanging onto me, this youngest son of mine had stepped up big time: flowers with notes on the proper occasions and a short phone chat every other day. *Every other day.* For a 28-year-old guy, this struck me as pretty amazing.

He's long been off the hook on that little gig, but I have all the roses he sent, dried and arranged in an antique planter, right where I see them during yoga every day.

And Herb, my husband. As I'd desperately wanted to hope from the beginning, this long walk through the valley of the shadow *had* turned out to be, yes, another in our long string of bad times we'd made it through together. The worst by far, we agree. But by the end, we had it figured out: I understood he was doing his very best, and he believed the same of me. What more could we ask of each other? In the living of all those nightmarish scenes, we'd finally found we had the power, together, to make sure that was not the way our story would end.

I knew I was well when, one promising spring morning, I walked out into the trees with my iPod set as usual to some murmuring healing track and suddenly had a thought: *I don't need this anymore.* I stopped, dug my iPod out of my Carhartts pocket and dialed up badass Bonnie Raitt.

That's more like it.

Welcome back.

All this time, while I'd been in some far, strange place, my small world had spun without me, whirling off changes—some unsettling, some reassuring.

People had moved. Eleanor had sold her house next to the Jackson Avenue bungalow, packed up and gone back to her beloved San Francisco. Never again would I experience the comfort of being welcomed to drop by and plop down on her sofa for a therapeutic heart-to-heart. Tess moved from Los Angeles back to her native Texas. Now, when I'd finally be well enough to go down with

Herb to see Aunt Catherine, there'd be no more walks in Hancock Park with this dearest of friends. No more lunches on the beach at Paradise Cove.

In Hawaii, Kona Village had closed forever. No going back.

Before I was well, the Jackson Avenue bungalow would change hands two more times and the white tile I'd agonized over would be ripped out for an enlargement of the bathroom. Someone posted a picture of the exterior on Pintarest, and people were sleuthing their way back to me for the exact color combination I'd used. My bungalow, it seemed, had become a little bit famous.

Before I was well, my mother had co-hosted a slew of deck parties at her new apartment and weathered hip replacement surgery without having to take more than a half-dozen tabs of Oxycodone.

Before I was well, Herb had managed to teach Ziwei to drive and she got her license.

Before I was well, the kids were all long settled into their new homes and jobs—Powell's Books, Lake Oswego Veterinary Emergency, 10 Barrel Brewing.

Amazing, that in the time it took my brain to heal, a child was conceived, born, and now follows his grampa around Wake Robin Farm, talking incessantly, saving his Chinese, of course, for conversations with his mother. At twenty-seven months, he may even have his daddy beat for precocious verbal skills. Will you forgive me? I am the most annoyingly braggy grandma ever, but I have to get this down for the record, the way this tiny construction site fan ran up to my mother and me in the backyard last week and crowed, "I've learned a new word. It's rotational hydraulic shears!"

I am not making this up. I couldn't. I always love real-life details better anyway.

As for me? Before I was well, I managed to drown my *fourth* cell phone in exactly the same manner as I'd killed the first three.

And I wrote this book.

Although perhaps it should have come as no surprise, it did strike me as such, the fact that when I rejoined the world, it turned out everyone else had aged the same three-and-a-half years I had. And people had not all necessarily been having a lovely picnic of it while I've been side-lined, either. The odd divorce loomed; some had received bad news by way of medical tests.

People had actually died—people in town my own age. Several writers, a gym buddy, a woman from an early moms group who'd brought her baby girl to roll around on a blanket in our backyard with baby Miles. Nothing quite like hearing that somebody actually *died* completely unexpectedly to give you pause and make you soberly glad that, whatever cards you've been dealt, you still get to play.

One day at the gym when I was finally making it back regularly, I looked at the hill through the wall of windows and thought one word: *Out.* I was out of my house, out of the darkness, out of the prison of illness and fatigue and isolation, out in the world.

I can't even express how good that felt.

Each time I go downtown now, I run into old friends and acquaintances.

"Wow, Linda," they invariably say, "haven't seen you in ages."

"Yeah, nobody has."

They laugh and ask if I've been on a trip. Well, sort of, but let's not go there.

"I've been pretty sick and sticking close to home, but I'm a lot better now. So, how are *you?*"

And it always seems like a small, quiet miracle each time I realize I don't necessarily have to launch into a sermon on the dangers of prescription drugs. Not right this minute anyway. My brain is no longer revved up, hard-wired into instant fight or flight. By some magic of regeneration, the alarm switch in there has finally been flipped to mute mode.

And what brought about this healing?

Time.

That's it.

That's all.

The simplest prescription and, also, the most difficult.

In Peter Thiele's recent book, *Zero to One,* he writes that a new idea is a truth in which you strongly believe, but may find yourself having trouble convincing *others* to believe.

Here's the new truth as I see it: In the prescribing of opioid painkillers and anti-anxiety benzodiazepines, the dictum *First, do no harm* is being broken by physicians every day. Your doctor may be the sweetest person alive, but he does not necessarily have your back. You must have your *own* back. You must accept the frightening truth that compliance to a doctor's prescription is no protection for your own precious brain. Your honest adherence to a pharmaceutical protocol that doesn't touch the official definition of abuse with a ten-foot pole will not save you. If you suspect you're in trouble because of your doctor's prescription, that doctor is probably the very last person who will want to hear about it.

If someone you love is going through this, try to be patient. Try to be kind. Hold that poor soul close. Read some material that helps explain what your loved one is struggling to endure. If the whole thing baffles you, remind yourself how lucky you are that it does. Please forgive them for their inability to adequately convey to you the true horror of their mental state. When they use the word hell, believe them.

If it's you, my friend, hang on.

Your miraculous brain wants to heal. It's trying. Have faith. Don't succumb to the temptation of an immediate but temporary fix of the very drugs that brought you to this point in the first place.

Feel free to borrow my script:

You're strong and brave, and if other people have made it through this, you can too.

Surely you're almost well, so don't you dare think of giving up.

Live through this and finally—please believe it—your suffering will be a thing of the past.

Hang tight to the knowledge that while you're down in the dark, we're up here rooting for you, and one of these days you'll be joining us, those who have escaped, finally, out into the light.

RESOURCES

>─────────────────<

Anatomy of an Epidemic: Magic Bullets, Psychiatric Drugs, and the Astonishing Rise of Mental Illness in America (Crown Publishing Group, 2010), Robert Whitaker. An eye-opening feat of investigative journalism, to be read cover to cover by anyone considering accepting a prescription for any sort of psych med for themselves or anyone they care about.

Recovery and Renewal: Your Essential Guide to Overcoming Dependency and Withdrawal from Sleeping Pills, Other "Benzo" Tranquillizers and Antidepressants (Jessica Kingsley Publishers, 2014), Baylissa Frederick. Amazingly comforting to read while in the deepest throes of benzo withdrawal, with a short, enlightening section to help caregivers understand what a person with PAWS is trying to endure.

Feeling Good: The New Mood Therapy (HarperCollins Publishing, Inc., 1999), David D. Burns, M. D. First published in 1980 and updated over the years, *Feeling Good* is the considered by many to be the gold standard in self help books on the subject of cognitive behavioral therapy.

Death Grip: a Climber's Escape from Benzo Madness (St. Martin's Press, 2013) Matt Samet. A well-written account of a young man's struggle to free himself from a tangled history of prescribed psych meds.

Total Recovery: Solving the Mystery of Chronic Pain and Depression (Rodale, 2013), Dr. Gary Kaplan, D.O. While not specifically about opioid or benzo withdrawal, I found these stories of people recovering from complex medical issues—often involving erroneous prescribing of meds—both inspiring and comforting.

A World of Hurt: Fixing Pain Medicine's Biggest Mistake (The New York Times Company, 2013), Barry Meier. A succinct explanation of why narcotic painkillers are not effective in treating chronic pain and the terrible consequences for those who were lead to believe they would be.

Spark! The Revolutionary New Science of Exercise and the Brain (Little, Brown and Company, 2008), John J. Ratey, MD. Perfect to read on a Kindle while pedaling your stationary bike. Even if you are already a fan of the power of exercise to improve your mood, it's reinforcing to understand the science behind it.

I Want to Change My Life: How to Overcome Anxiety, Depression & Addiction (Modern Therapies, 2010), Steven M. Melemis, Ph.D. M.D. The first place I found acknowledgment of the long range symptoms of post acute withdrawal syndrome, although at least in this book, the author does not deal with addiction by prescription.

The Body Keeps the Score: Brain, Mind, and Body in the Healing of Trauma (Penguin Books, 2014) Bessel A. van der Kolk, M. D. Great explanation of how emotional trauma can translate into physical pain and illness.

In the Realm of Hungry Ghosts, Close Encounters with Addiction (North Atlantic Books, 2010, originally by Alfred A. Knopf Canada, 2008), Gabor Mate, M.D. A doctor's amazingly compassionate examination of the lives and compromised brains of those suffering from addiction.

Cure: a Journey into the Science of Mind Over Body (Crown Publishers, 2016), Jo Marchant. A clear-eyed exploration of the extent to which we might hope positive thinking could help us.

A Meditation for Help with ANGER & FORGIVENESS (www.healthjourneys.com), Belleruth Naparstek.

Music to Inspire Positive Thinking, Scientifically designed by Dr. Lee R. Bartel to boost alpha and beta brainwave activity. Somerset Entertainment Ltd., 2009. I don't understand how this works, but I'm convinced it does and I'm hooked on my CD.

Benzo Buddies—support for people wanting to get off of benzodiazepines. www.benzobuddies.org.

Physicians for Responsible Opioid Prescribing—physicians trying to inform patients and their physicians about the hazards of narcotic pain medications. www.supportprop.org

Mad in America. Science, Psychiatry and Community. www.madinamerica.com

Beyond Meds: everything matters—Monica Cassani's award-winning web magazine featuring resources for those wanting to get off of psych meds. https://beyondmeds.com.

ACKNOWLEDGMENTS

Because my healing was pretty much a Little Red Hen project, it seems fitting that the publishing of this book would be as well, which means I have no lengthy list of agents and editors to thank, or even my usual first readers. For the most part, the people who were there for me already appear in these pages.

I do want to thank my childhood Bluebird buddy, Susie Nieto, who, when I was finally able to explain why I couldn't take her up on her gracious offer to come hang in Hood River for hiking and sailboarding, mounted a faithful campaign of weekly check-in calls that often came just when I needed a voice from the outside world the most.

My cousin, Heidi Sivers-Boyce, likewise provided affectionate and continuing support by way of her thoughtful emails.

Registered nurse and masseuse, Mya English, allowed me to vent as she did what she could to help with the healing power of touch.

Certain people unknowingly shot rays of light into my darkness during this time by writing to me about my previously published books. Henry Wadsworth Longfellow wrote: *Give what you have to give. To someone it may be worth more than you dare think.* Good words to live by, I've always thought, and that's what happened here. These people gave, and it meant more to me than they could possibly have realized.

Sometimes, for me, a book has an angel, and on this one that title goes to my dear friend Theresa Nelson Cooney. She not only held onto me during my struggle to heal, she also served as my first reader. No one else in my life can take a manuscript of mine and scribble it up with the exuberant and encouraging hearts, stars and exclamation points she knows the third-grader in me still needs. Tess, I'm so glad you're in this world.

I'm not sure how my story might have gone had I not eventually connected with my friends on the BenzoBuddies board, the club none of us wanted to be in, but were so glad to find. I'm indebted in particular to the folks who PMed me with encouragement and support for my posts. You know who you are. Your kind words helped and, along with everything else, will be remembered.

Lastly, I'd like to thank the Authors Guild for all it does to try to protect the laws of copyright and the livelihoods of professional writers in the current internet "sharing economy."

Also by Linda Crew

Children of the River

Someday I'll Laugh About This

Nekomah Creek

Ordinary Miracles

Nekomah Creek Christmas

Fire on the Wind

Long Time Passing

Brides of Eden: a True Story Imagined

A Heart for Any Fate: Westward to Oregon 1845